MACRO DIET COOKBOOK

Supercharge Fat Loss,
Boost Energy and Build Muscle
Without Giving Up Your Favorite Foods

100 Healthy & Easy Recipes,
Flexible Meal Plans,
Beginners guide to counting your macros

Michael Smith

Table of Contents

FREE BONUS MATERIAL

Thank you for reading this book. I hope you find it insightful, inspiring, and practical and I hope it helps you build that strong and healthy body you really desire.

To help you get the best results as fast as possible I've put together additional free resources:

- **Macro Friendly Grocery List** to never run out of ideas what to eat
- **6 Step Quick Start Guide** to finally take your fitness under control
- **Daily Checklist** to stay on track with your fitness goals
- **Example Meal Plan** to supercharge your fat loss
- **Comprehensive Workout Log Sheet** for keeping track of your workouts
- **Top Tips for Seniors** to enjoy your life and avoid health problems as you age

To get your bonuses go to:
http://bit.ly/4oMJRRK

or scan QR code with your camera

Introduction

"It is health that is the real wealth and not pieces of gold and silver."

Mahatma Gandhi

Lose weight and stay fit without giving up on the foods you love! Does this sound dubious? Chances are you are imagining eating extremely small portions and severe calorie restrictions when you think about diet. Most conventional diets are based on these notions. Well, you are in for a treat because the macro diet is unlike any other diet you have ever come across.

You've probably heard the saying, "health is wealth." Turns out, this is quite true. A healthy body is perhaps the most important thing anyone can possess. When you are physically healthy, it gives you the energy needed to chase your goals and live the life you desire. The simplest way to ensure your health is to pay attention to your diet. Your diet plays a bigger role in your overall well-being than you have probably ever even thought of. A healthy diet is not synonymous with bland food. It certainly doesn't mean you need to eat extremely small portions or starve yourself. Instead, a healthy and wholesome diet includes ingredients filled with nutrients that your body requires for its overall health and well-being. A healthy diet is devoid of junk food and replaces it with healthier options. When you combine this with exercise, improving your overall health automatically becomes easier.

These days, there are a variety of dietary protocols to choose from. They each have their pros and cons. Whether it is fat loss or weight loss and its maintenance there are different diets to choose from. When there are so many options available, it can be quite confusing and overwhelming to pick one. Well, you can stop your search here, because the macro diet is one of the best diets available these days. Or maybe you have tried different diets but nothing seems to be working. Some diets can be extremely restrictive too. A common reason why most prematurely give up on their diet is that it restricts their favorite foods or prescribes bland and measly portions. If you have experienced these struggles and are looking for a healthier and sustainable eating pattern, the macro diet is all you need.

The macro diet, as the name suggests, focuses on the macronutrients your body requires. Carbohydrates, proteins, and fats are the three macros your body requires for its health and functioning. There is no one-die-fits-all approach when it comes to eating healthily. Instead, you need to take into consideration different factors that are at play such as your usual lifestyle, time available, or the goals you want to achieve. You should also understand that your body's nutritional needs are different and you are unique. The macro diet caters to this basic difference. This diet makes you aware of your existing level of nutrition and any imbalances in it. It holds you accountable and makes sure you are consuming the right quantity of food. It makes you aware of the actual serving sizes and ensures you aren't deprived of your favorite foods. Also, it is incredibly easy to follow because the protocols it prescribes are practical and sustainable.

Once you start following this diet, your life will become easier. There'll be a positive change in your overall health and fitness levels. Whether you want to lose weight or build lean muscle there are a lot of benefits this diet offers. Any fitness or health goal you have can be attained with this diet. Are you wondering how I know all this? Well, I believe it is time for a little introduction.

Hello, my name is Michael Smith. I was your typical average man who was trying to keep together his family, and job and make the most of my life. One fine day, something just seemed to click. As I reached my midlife, I started worrying that I would never feel or look the way I used to. This was when I decided it was time to dive deep into the world of fitness, health, and nutrition. This marked the beginning of intensive research and study to understand the answer to all the questions I had. Over the years, I managed to combine my passion for research with personal positive experiences by making simple changes to my diary routine. I realized the importance of nutrition and focusing on eating the right foods. It's not just about foods that are considered to be healthy. Instead, I realized I need to work along with my body's metabolism and cater to its nutritional needs and requirements. This proved to be the missing piece of the puzzle. Implementing this newfound knowledge I realized I can improve my overall health while catering to my body's nutritional needs and requirements. This diet also enabled me to help achieve my fitness objectives.

Now, I believe that even you can benefit from the years I spent researching and testing different facets of health and nutrition. I have created a step-by-step and realistic road map that will help achieve your weight loss and fitness goals. It will also help with any age-related health problems and make you feel better than you ever did. I believe my passion and research about leading a healthier life will prove beneficial for you as well.

This book will act as your guide every step of the way. It is filled with helpful and practical information that can be easily implemented into your daily life. You don't have to compromise on any aspect of your life for the sake of health and wellbeing. Instead, this diet works in tandem with all of the facets of your usual life.

Apart from this, you will also be introduced to a variety of macro diet-friendly recipes. You don't have to spend hours together in the kitchen cooking nutritious meals. Instead, these simple recipes will make cooking a breeze. You can rest easy knowing that the delicious meals you are eating cater to your body's nutritional needs and requirements. You will also be introduced to different steps to be followed to calculate the total macros you should eat, their importance on your overall health, and calculating your daily calories. Once you are armed with all this information and the sample meal plans provided in this book, you can eat your way to a healthier and fitter life. Put together a meal plan using the suggestions given in this book. After this, stock your pantry with the ingredients needed and follow the simple recipes. Yes, this is about it!

So, are you eager to learn more about all those? If yes, there is no time like the present to get started!

Chapter 1: What Is the Macro Diet?

"Healthy eating is a way of life, so it's important to establish routines that are simple, realistically, and ultimately livable."

Horace

Do you want to shift to a healthy and wholesome diet that is easy to follow? Do you want to achieve your weight loss and fitness goals without sacrificing the foods you love and enjoy? Do you want a diet that is sustainable in the long run? Do you want to do all this but don't know where to start? If yes, the macro diet is perfect for you!

The macro diet is steadily gaining popularity in the fitness and health circles and for all the right reasons. This diet is also known as IIFYM (If It Fits Your Macros) or flexible dieting. It is about focusing on consuming the macronutrients your body requires. The three macronutrients you require for maintaining your overall health and fitness are carbohydrates, fats, and proteins. This diet does not cut out any specific food group. It simply makes you aware of your body's needs and requirements. Depending on your health or fitness objectives, the diet you follow will also differ. Most conventional diets do not offer room for customization. Given that we all have varying goals and our bodies function differently, a conventional diet might not offer the right dietary guidelines. Unlike conventional diets, the macro diet offers basic guidelines that can be used to create a highly-customized diet as per your needs and requirements.

Benefits of the Macro Diet

Here are all the different benefits associated with the macro diet.

Understanding What You're Eating and Prevent Nutrient Deficiencies

You might have come across the saying, "You are what you eat." I believe the diet you follow affects every aspect of your life. It's not just your weight or fat percentage but it influences how you feel as well. When you can see the impact of food choices you make on your health, the inclination to make better choices increases.

This is perhaps one of the coolest aspects of counting macros. It gives you better insight into the nutritional content of the foods you eat. Most of us eat a variety of food items without even considering our nutritional profile. When you need to track macros, you are forced to pay attention to this. Whether it is purchasing a packet of chips or ordering take-out, you become conscious of the macros present in each of them.

After all, the goal of this diet is to ensure you are consuming macronutrients as per your body's needs and requirements in synchronization with the goals you wish to achieve. The macro diet encourages healthy decision-making, especially in terms of the foods you eat and their portion size. This information also gives better insight into understanding your body's satiety and hunger levels. When all these factors are put together, it becomes easy to see how the macro diet promotes healthier eating choices.

Better Energy Levels

A common problem with most regular diets is they usually restrict the consumption of specific food groups. Doing this is undesirable because it can drain your energy. You cannot maintain your energy levels or improve them unless you consume all the macros (Alicia L Carreiro *et al.*, 2016). And the macros diet enables you to do this in a balanced way. For instance, a high-fat diet cuts out all carbs. Since carbs are the primary source of energy, cutting them out is unhelpful. So, the macro diet works because it works along with your body. By balancing the number of carbs, proteins, and fats you consume, you can achieve your fitness and health goals. You can also do this without getting tired.

Improved Sleep

Have you ever struggled to fall asleep after eating an extremely large meal at night? Well, this is because there is a direct relationship between the diet you follow and your quality of sleep (Marie-Pierre St-Onge *et al.*, 2016). This is because such heavy meals take a long time to be digested. Usually, meals that are sleep-friendly include plenty of fruits and vegetables, whole grains, lean protein, and dairy. Portion size along with quality are crucial factors. By limiting the consumption of processed foods and replacing them with wholesome and unprocessed ingredients, you are not only improving your health but your ability to sleep through the night too. By following the macro diet, you can catch up on some much-needed rest.

Quality Control

Counting macros is a great way to focus on the quality of food you are consuming. Instead of mentally sorting through items and categorizing them as healthy or unhealthy, tracking macros enables you to exactly see what you are eating. Instead of merely labeling junk food as unhealthy, counting macros enables you to see why they are unhealthy. For instance, you probably know that eating a donut is not good. When you start tracking macros, you will realize the astounding amount of carbs and fat present in it instead of simply thinking of it as the enemy. It consciously teaches you to pick nutrient-dense foods instead of making them feel like a forced choice. Also, reducing the consumption of junk and unhealthy foods such as chips, sweetened beverages, processed meats, and so on results in weight gain (Dariush Mozaffarian *et al.*, 2011).

Promotes Accountability

Accountability is needed in all aspects of life and the diet you follow is not an exception. Have you ever started a diet but given up on it prematurely? Or maybe you follow a diet for a couple of weeks or even months only to revert to unhealthy eating patterns? Maybe you started exercising but couldn't follow through with the schedule you created? When you understand that you are the only one accountable for the food choices you make and your health, your attitude toward the diet also changes for the better. Tracking what you eat promotes your ability to lose weight and maintain it (John Spencer Ingels *et al.*, 2017).

Once you start counting or tracking your macros, you'll be surprised by the number of carbs or fats you are consuming. When you can see the exact number of macros present in the foods you opt for, your sense of accountability increases. Once you realize that you are the only one responsible for the choices you make, you'll feel more in control of yourself. Well, this logic is quite similar to the one used in the world of business, "If you don't track it, you can't improve it." After all, how can you know there is any scope for change or improvement, without being aware of the current situation? So, if you want to eat healthier or follow the macro diet, then you must become aware of the food choices you make. This is what the macro diet does.

It Is Flexible

What is the first thing that pops into your head when you hear the word diet? You might start worrying about giving up on the foods you love and enjoy. Whether it is mac and cheese or fish fingers, you probably have different comfort foods. The thought of not being able to eat such foods because of the diet can be frustrating. It can also become a source of stress.

This diet is not restrictive by any means. Instead of worrying about giving up on the foods you love, it encourages you to pay attention to the macros in them. As long as the food you're eating fits the desired macro ratio or proportion, it is all good. Doesn't it make dieting more fun and exciting?

It Is Satisfying

When you start counting macros and stick to the limit, it is nothing short of an achievement. These personal achievements add up and become an extremely powerful motivator that helps achieve your weight loss or fitness objectives. Regardless of the goal, you have set for yourself, you can achieve it once you start counting and tracking macros. When you see yourself hit the daily target of macros and consistently do so, it increases your confidence in yourself. It will also increase your motivation to stick to the diet.

Customization

There are no hard and fast rules about what you can and cannot on this diet. The primary focus is to track the macros you are consuming and ensure you stick to the daily limits. This diet is beneficial because it offers a greater degree of customization. Depending on the goals you wish to attain, the macros you consume can also be changed. For instance, macros required for weight loss will be different from the ones associated with developing and maintaining lean muscle. By factoring in different needs and requirements as per your goals, this diet offers plenty of flexibility.

Some Concerns

Even though the macro diet is flexible and perfectly customizable, one thing you shouldn't forget is it is still a diet. it is not something you can start one day and expect miraculous results overnight. Instead, it requires commitment and conscious effort. To ensure you stick to the diet and avoid giving up on it, developing self-motivation and discipline are needed. The good news is, once you start paying attention to the calories you are consuming and consciously make healthy food choices, both motivation and discipline increase. Since it is a diet, ensure that you consult your healthcare provider or physician before making a change, especially if you have any existing health conditions.

Do not use this diet as an excuse to binge on unhealthy foods. don't fool yourself into thinking that you simply need to stick to a daily calorie intake. you will learn in detail about the important aspects of nutrition prescribed by this diet in the subsequent chapters.

The primary focus of this diet is on the macronutrients you obtain. That said, other micronutrients such as minerals and vitamins are equally important. Without them, your body doesn't get its daily dose of nourishment. To ensure you overcome this drawback of the macro diet, don't forget about considering your micronutrient intake. If needed, you can add a multivitamin supplement after consulting your healthcare provider.

The macro diet is easy to follow but it is not ideal for those with specific health conditions. Once again, consult your healthcare provider. Similarly, those who are recovering from an eating disorder or have a history of eating disorders, should not attempt any diet. Unless you have fully recovered, sticking to a diet increases the risk of relapse.

Key Takeaway

- The macro diet is not only simple to follow but sustainable too.

- It is based on the concept of tracking macros instead of obsessing over portions consumed or restricting certain food groups.

- Following the macro diet will increase your sense of accountability, promote healthier eating habits and choices, offer customization options, and is inclusive.

Chapter 2: Understanding the Main Food Groups

"Health is a relationship between you and your body."

Terri Guillemets

Following any diet becomes easy once you are aware of all that it entails. The macro diet, as the name suggests, is based on the macronutrients you are consuming. Understanding what macronutrients are and their importance will make it easier to see why you must focus on them.

What Are Macros?

Macronutrients are commonly known as macros and they are essential nutrients your body requires to stay healthy. As the name suggests, these nutrients are needed in large quantities to ensure optimal bodily functions. They give the maximum amount of energy from the food consumed. The three macronutrients are carbohydrates, proteins, and fats. Each of these macros also contains different calories. Carbohydrates and proteins contain 4 calories per gram whereas fat contains 9 calories per gram.

Carbohydrates

Almost every piece of food you consume has carbohydrates and therefore, they are the most significant energy source for your body. The level of carbohydrates is different in different foods.

Usually, a typical western diet is rich in carbs and sugars. The problem with them is they are the leading cause of weight and fat gain. Yes, it is not fats but carbs that are the primary culprit. Even though they aren't as important as proteins or fats, removing them isn't ideal. This is because they are the primary source of glucose, which is the body's go-to source for energy generation. Once your body has fulfilled its energy requirements from glucose, the remainder is stored in the form of bundles known as glycogen. Glycogen is stored in the liver and muscles. The space available in them is limited and once it is full, the extra glucose is stored in the form of fats. Over a period, when left unregulated, this results in fat and weight gain. Some carb-restricting diets such as the ketogenic diet or Atkins might offer good results but eliminating them altogether isn't a good idea.

This is because your body is used to obtaining energy from them. Even if it doesn't seem like much to you, severe carb restriction is a significant challenge for your body and mind. Also, foods rich in carbs taste quite good and are known to improve the mood by triggering the production of a neurotransmitter known as serotonin. So, cutting them out can result in extreme mood swings. Instead, if you just become mindful of the type of carbs you consume, it will be better for your health and fitness goals. The two major forms of carbohydrates are monosaccharides and polysaccharides. Their chemical structure is the only difference between them. Monosaccharides are simple carbohydrates, and they are also known as sugars. Common examples of simple carbs include baked treats, sodas, breakfast cereal, fruit juices, and most prepackaged and junk food. When compared to monosaccharides, polysaccharides are more abundant in a variety of foods. They are also known as complex carbohydrates. Some examples of complex carbs include whole grains, fruits and vegetables rich in fiber, and beans.

Some common and healthy sources of carbohydrates are as follows:

- all varieties of beans

- bananas

- blueberries

- bread

- oatmeal

- oats

- pasta

- potatoes

- quinoa

- rice

- wheat

The carbohydrates you consume are broken down into glucose which is the primary source of energy. Some specific organs including the brain require glucose to function efficiently. Glucose can also be synthesized from proteins depending on your body's necessity through a process known as gluconeogenesis. Carbohydrates also help synthesize certain amino acids that act as building blocks of cells.

Fiber is also a type of carbohydrate that is not broken down in the gastrointestinal tract or the GI tract. This, in turn, ensures consistent bowel movements and keeps the intestinal tract healthy. Common sources of fiber include broccoli, berries, whole grains, leafy vegetables, nuts and seeds, oatmeal, whole-wheat products, fruits with edible skins, and beans. These fiber-rich foods don't cause any fluctuations in blood sugar levels unlike simple carbs. It is better to avoid processed or simple carbohydrates because they are easily digested by the body. They release glucose quickly, resulting in fluctuations in blood sugar levels.

Fluctuations in blood sugar level are undesirable because when left unregulated they become a risk factor for a variety of chronic health conditions. Such fluctuations in blood sugar are also associated with weight gain. Whenever you eat, insulin is produced by the pancreas. Insulin is a hormone that enables your body to utilize the energy obtained from food consumed. It does this by unlocking the cells so the glucose can enter them and fulfill their energy needs. The problem starts when the cells become resistant to this hormone. A simple analogy to understand this relationship is to think of your body as a vehicle. If the vehicle is carrying a load of 500 lbs then it increases the energy needed to function. It requires more gas and over a period, the engine is worn-out due to the greater stress on it to obtain the required performance. Insulin is the gas line running between the engine and the fuel tank. It becomes harder to obtain the fuel when insulin resistance is squeezing this line.

It is difficult for the insulin resistant cells to utilize the glucose available. Over a period, this results in buildup of blood sugar levels resulting in weight gain. This is because the high levels of blood sugar signal the pancreas to produce more insulin. But all this insulin isn't being utilized. Instead, the body takes this insulin available as a signal to store more fats instead of using it as energy. The relationship between blood sugar and weight gain is a vicious cycle where one factor feeds and propagates the other

Proteins

Protein is needed for the growth and development of tissues in the body. It is also needed for repairing and protecting lean muscle mass. Protein is essentially made of amino acids. Amino acids are of two types and they are nonessential and essential amino acids. Non-essential amino acids don't have to be consumed through the diet because your body can make them. On the other hand, essential amino acids are not produced within and must be obtained from dietary sources. In some cases, essential amino acids are also transformed into non-essential ones depending on your body's needs and requirements.

Ensure that you consume sufficient protein because it is known to reduce your appetite and manage hunger levels. Protein is by far the most filling when compared to other macros. When you eat sufficient protein, it reduces the production of a hunger-inducing hormone known as ghrelin which reduces the urge to eat. This, in turn, promotes weight loss and maintenance. It is also needed for improving muscle mass and strength. Since protein is the building block of muscles, consuming sufficient protein is needed.

Protein is also needed for maintaining bone health, reducing cravings, and improving metabolism. The thermic effect of protein is higher than that of carbs. The thermic effect essentially refers to the calories your body spends to digest and utilize the nutrients present in the food consumed. When you eat sufficient protein, your body metabolism gets a boost and it promotes fat burning. Since protein is a building block of all tissues and organs, it promotes internal repair and healing, especially after injuries.

Protein is helpful but balance is needed. Consuming too much protein is not good for your health and wellbeing. Understand that eating bigger portions of steak doesn't equate to bigger muscles or quick weight loss. Once your daily quota of protein is met, the excess is stored in the form of fat cells. The excess calories are always stored as fat. So, eating extra protein increases the levels of blood lipids and the risk of cardiovascular disorders as well. Excess protein can be taxing on the kidneys, especially in those with existing kidney disease or problems.

As per the dietary requirements, anywhere between 10–35% of your daily calories must be from protein. A common idea most have about protein consumption is to have 1 gram of protein per pound of bodyweight. This is a simple way to calculate but it is a misconception. Excessive protein intake for an average individual is when you eat more than 2 grams per kilogram or 0.9 grams per pound of your body weight (Wempen, 2022). So, one gram of protein per pound of bodyweight is excess protein for non-professional sportspersons. Due to this, the ideal method, according to American College of Sports Medicine, to calculate your protein requirement is to consume 1.2–1.7 grams of protein per kilogram of your body weight. This translates to 0.5–0.8 grams per pound of body weight per day as protein intake. Hitting this protein target is vital, especially if you are over 40 years old or lift weights regularly. For instance, if someone weighs 200 lbs., then their protein intake must be between 100 and 160 grams per day. Stick to this protein limit if you are not going to be a professional bodybuilder because this level of intake is sufficient to increase muscle mass in combination with physical activity.

Another common mistake most make is they believe one piece of chicken breast (4 oz or 122 grams size) is equivalent to 122 grams of protein. This is untrue and around 4 oz of chicken contains 20 grams of protein. So, if a 200 lbs individual needs 120 grams of protein, then they will need about six pieces of 4 oz each chicken breast or alternative protein sources.

Some healthy sources of protein your body needs are as follows:

- dairy products

- eggs

- fish and seafood

- legumes

- meat

- nuts

- whey protein

Fats

Fats are commonly demonized and considered to be the enemy of health. Unsurprisingly a lot of people are scared of fats. Well, it is time to change how you feel about fats because all fats are not harmful. Fats or lipids can be either solid or liquid. They are commonly categorized as trans fats, saturated fats, and unsaturated fats. Fats enable your body to store energy, produce certain hormones, and absorb fat-soluble vitamins. It also maintains the integrity of cellular membranes and cushions organs. Let's look at the different types of fats.

Trans fats should be eliminated from your diet if you want to improve your overall health and well-being. These are commonly present in hydrogenated oils. Whenever hydrogen molecules are added to unsaturated fats, it results in the production of trans fats. Margarine, baked goods, fried foods, and even shortening include these harmful fats and you must avoid them at all costs.

Saturated fats are healthy in limited amounts. However, excess consumption of saturated fats increases levels of harmful cholesterol along with that cardiovascular disorders. Consuming a moderate amount of saturated fats is needed for maintaining your overall health. The most common sources of saturated fats are animal foods such as fatty beef, pork, poultry with skin, cream, butter, full-fat dairy products, and lamb. Around 5–6% of your daily calories should be from saturated fats and no more as per the recommendations of the American Heart Association.

The healthiest type of fats are the unsaturated variants. They are usually found in a liquid state at room temperature and are needed for regulating your body's metabolism. They also help maintain the elasticity of cell membranes, promote blood flow in the body, and are needed for the growth and regeneration of cells. They also contain essential omega-3 and omega-6 fatty acids that are good for your health. Consuming plenty of omega-3 fatty acids is needed for stabilizing heart health, reducing the risk of cardiovascular disorders, tackling inflammation, and promoting internal healing. The most common sources of these healthy fats include

- avocados and their oil

- naturally fatty fish such as salmon, mackerel, and tuna

- nuts and nut-based butter

- olive and olive oil

- seeds

Understanding the different types of fats is needed, certain types of fat are good while others are not. Stay away from trans fats and certain types of saturated fats to ensure your overall health and well-being. The ideal requirement of fats is 0.2–0.5 grams per pound of body weight per day. According to the U.S Department of Agriculture and U.S. Department of Health and Human Services the daily intake of calories should be 20% to 35% from fat (Dietary Guidelines for Americans, 2020-2025. 9th edition, December 2020).

Are Calories Important?

You might have heard the term calories tossed around in regular conversations. However, do you know what it means? Calories are nothing but a unit of energy your body requires and utilizes as fuel. Most diets usually reduce one or more of the macronutrients to promote weight loss. Well, eliminating a specific macronutrient does more harm than good. Instead, it is better to focus on the calories you are consuming to ensure you can follow the macro diet.

We all require calories to survive. Different factors determine your calorie requirement. The most important factor is your level of physical activity. The calorie consumption of a professional athlete will be different from someone leading a sedentary lifestyle. Calorie requirement is also based on your age. Usually, the calories required by a younger person are greater than that of an older one.

A calorie deficit is needed for weight loss. To do this, you'll need to consume fewer calories than your body is utilizing. A simple way to increase the calories your body utilizes is by moving more. Another great way is to reduce your calorie intake. By combining these ideas, you can easily attain your weight loss, fitness, or any other health objective.

Considerations

If you want to make the most of the benefits offered by the macro diet, then paying attention to the food choices you make is needed. It's not just about following the daily macro requirement. It's also about ensuring you are consuming nutrient-dense ingredients that offer nourishment to your body. Staying away from sugar and calorie-rich beverages, trans fats, white flour, and processed food is needed for improving your overall health. All these ingredients mentioned here trigger inflammation, increase blood sugar levels, resulting in clogged arteries and increases the risk of a variety of chronic health problems. Eating too many of these ingredients will only worsen your current state of health. Apart from all these benefits, cutting back on sugar and other above-mentioned foods make it easier to achieve your weight loss goals too.

The simplest way to stick to this diet is by following the 80/20 rule. This rule simply suggests that you need to ensure at least 80% of your daily calories are from whole and unprocessed foods and the rest can include all the food items that you like. Whether it is ice cream, a packet of chips, or any other guilty pleasure, you can still eat what you like provided you consume your daily share of healthy calories. When you fill-up on 80% of unprocessed food, the chances of binging on unhealthy foods also reduce. Following the macro diet is simple because it does not restrict any food groups and instead, it offers the information needed to make healthy food choices.

Key Takeaways

- Macronutrients or macros are essential nutrients that account for a significant percentage of your daily energy requirement.

- The three macros your body requires for optimal health and functioning are proteins, fats, and carbohydrates.

- A well-balanced diet is a perfect combination of macros.

- Even though the macro diet doesn't promote obsessive calorie counting, paying attention to the source of calories is needed.

Chapter 3: How to Figure out

Your Macros?

"Take care of your body. It's the only place you have to live."

Jim Rohn

Now that you are aware of the macros and their importance, it is time to learn about the macro diet. To follow this diet, you must determine how many macros you need to consume.

Fat loss and weight loss are the most common goals of those interested in the macro diet. Before doing this, you must understand the basic nutritional principle of calories in and calories out. Calories are a unit of energy. From a nutritional perspective, calories are the energy derived whenever you eat or drink anything. This is then used to sustain physical activity and bodily functions. Do you remember the concept of a calorie deficit that you were introduced to in the previous chapter? It occurs when your body utilizes more calories than you consume. Whenever you eat, a certain number of calories go into your body. On the other hand, when you exercise or engage in any physical activity, calories are utilized. Your body also utilizes calories for its maintenance functions such as respiration, digestion, and so on. Weight gain occurs when calorie consumption is greater than utilization. On the other hand, if you want to lose weight, you will obviously need to increase calorie expenditure instead of consumption. This is the basic principle that you need to use for manipulating your body weight as well as composition. Reducing your calorie intake, increasing physical activity, or doing both will result in a calorie deficit. That said, the deficit shouldn't be drastic because severe calorie restriction is unhealthy. You will learn about this in the next section.

Before moving on to learning about counting macros, an interesting fact is that a pound of fat has around 3,500 calories. Well, that is a lot of calories. Now, you needn't worry too much about the number, but it gives you a starting point to understand how many calories you will need to consume.

Calorie Requirements for Maintenance

The first step in understanding how many calories your body requires is to determine your maintenance calories. The energy your body requires for its course needs is your maintenance calories. To determine your maintenance calories, let's start with your body weight. You will need to consume 14–16 calories per lb. of your body weight. There are multiple formulas you can use to calculate the maintenance calories. You can also use online calculators for this purpose. However, simplicity is always better. A simple means to calculate your maintenance calories to understand how to manipulate daily macros is to stick to the 14–16 limit. If you lead a sedentary lifestyle then opt for the lower need of the scale, which is 14 calories per lb. of bodyweight. Women need to opt for the same range— 14 calories per lb. of bodyweight. On the other hand, if you are active and exercise regularly, opt for the higher limit of 16 calories per lb. of body weight.

Weight in pounds	How Many Calories You Need Per Day		
	Lower end	Average	Higher end
100	1,400	1,500	1,600
110	1,540	1,650	1,760
120	1,680	1,800	1,920
130	1,820	1,950	2,080
140	1,960	2,100	2,240
150	2,100	2,250	2,400
160	2,240	2,400	2,560
170	2,380	2,550	2,720
180	2,520	2,700	2,880
190	2,660	2,850	3,040
200	2,800	3,000	3,360

210	2,940	3,150	3,520
220	3,080	3,300	3,680
230	3,220	3,450	3,680
240	3,360	3,600	3,840
250	3,500	3,750	4,000

Let's use an example to make things easier. Adam weighs 200 lbs. and leads a moderately active lifestyle. To make the calculation easy, let's assume he needs 15 calories per lb. for maintenance. So, Adam's maintenance calories are 200 lbs. x 15 calories, which gives us 3,000 calories. It means he needs to consume 3,000 calories daily for maintenance.

Calorie Requirements for Weight Loss

Now, let's use the maintenance calories to determine his calorie deficit for weight loss. By subtracting 500 calories per day from his daily intake, you get 2,500 calories. The deficit to be maintained is 500 calories. If he maintains this deficit for a week, it results in a calorie loss of 3,500. Does this number sound familiar? Well, it is the same number of calories that are present in a pound of fat. So, if he consumes 2,500 calories daily and maintains this for a week, it will result in a fat loss of one pound! You don't need a calorie restriction of more than 500 calories per day or 25% of daily quota for healthy weight loss (*Bigger Leaner Stronger*, Michael Mathews, 2019).

You simply need to subtract 500 calories from your daily maintenance calories for a calorie deficit. So, a 160 lbs woman will need 2,240 calories daily and this is her maintenance calories. For fat loss, she needs to subtract 500 from 2,240 daily calories. The number of calories she needs to consume daily for fat loss will be 1,740! One thing you must remember is this isn't an exact science. A variety of factors are at play that influences your body's ability to lose fat. These factors include water weight, hormones, and any fluctuations of sodium and glycogen. So, don't be disheartened if it doesn't result in an exact fat loss of one pound by the end of the week. On the whole, following these calorie limits will promote fat loss.

Calculating Macros

The Acceptable Macronutrient Distribution as per the Dietary Guidelines for Americans is 20–35% of daily calories from fats, 10–35% of calories from proteins, and 45–65% of calories from carbohydrates. Once you are aware of the macros you need and the calories you consume, it is time to do a little math. The three steps you must follow are:

- Determine the total calorie requirement.

- Determine your requirements for essential macros: protein and fat

- Determine how much carbs you will need to collect remaining calories

Let's go back to Adam's example to get a better understanding of this process. Now, for calculating the macros, it is time to determine the calories for each of the macros. Here is a quick recap of the caloric value of the three macros.

- Fat–9 calories per gram

- Carbs–4 calories per gram

- Protein–4 calories per gram

The ideal macronutrient requirement is as follows:

- 0.5–0.8 grams of protein per pound of bodyweight.

- 0.2–0.5 grams of fat per pound of body weight.

- The rest of the daily calories available will be from carbohydrates.

As mentioned previously, Adam's daily calorie intake will be 2,500. Using the information given above, it is time to determine his macro requirements. His average protein requirement is 0.8 grams per pound, the fat requirement is 0.35 grams per pound and the rest is allocated for carbs. Now, using this information, we get the following macros for Adam. The final step of determining the daily macros is to convert the number of proteins, fats, and carbs into grams.

Protein Requirement

To obtain the protein breakdown, multiply bodyweight by the ideal range of proteins that was given above.

200 x 0.8 = 160 grams of protein

So, the number of calories to be obtained from protein is

160 grams x 4 = 640 calories

Fat Requirement

To obtain the fat breakdown, multiply body weight by the ideal range of fats that was given above.

200 x 0.35 = 70 grams of fat

So, the number of calories to be obtained from fat is

70 grams x 9 = 630 calories

Carbohydrate Requirement

To determine the carb requirement, merely add the daily calories from fats and protein and subtract their combined figure from the target calories. For instance, in Adam's case, his daily calorie limit is 2,500. From this, 640 calories are obtained from protein and 630 calories from fats. The remaining calories are obtained from carbs. So, his carb requirement is 1,230 calories per day (2,500 - 640 - 630 = 1,230 calories). Once you have this number, it is time to convert the calories into grams. Each gram of carb has four calories. So, to obtain 1,230 calories from carbs, he will need to consume around 308 grams of carbs.

If you take a moment and look at these simple calculations, you will realize that the macro proportions in percentages (50% from carbs, and 25% each from fats and proteins) perfectly meets the recommendations of acceptable macronutrient distribution ranges (AMDR). Per Dietary Guidelines for Americans by the U.S Department of Agriculture and U.S. Department of Health and Human Services AMDR for people's daily intake of calories are: 45% to 65% from carbs, 10% to 35% from protein, 20% to 35% from fat (Dietary Guidelines for Americans, 2020-2025. 9th edition, December 2020). Following this macros breakdown is needed for supporting tissue growth, facilitating energy production, and avoiding any potential nutrient deficiencies and associated problems. The meal plans that you will be introduced to later on in this book are based on the above-mentioned guidelines.

Calorie Requirements for Building Muscle

You were already introduced to the macros calculation for maintenance and fat loss. Now, the next fitness goal we can focus on is weight gain or muscle building. By now you would have realized that calculating macros is not a difficult process by any means.

The only thing you need to remember when it comes to weight gain and muscle building is to increase your calorie consumption. Previously, you were introduced to the concept of calorie deficit wherein your body's calorie expenditure was greater than the consumption. The opposite of this is a calorie surplus. It occurs when calorie consumption is more than expenditure. You need a 10% calorie surplus over your maintenance calories to achieve this goal. For instance, if your maintenance calories are 3,000 per day, then the surplus to be maintained is 10% of this. It gives you an additional 300 calories. This means the total calories to be consumed for weight gain and muscle building are 3,300 calories per day.

Let's use an example to get a better understanding. Henry is a 200 lbs. man and needs around 3,000 calories daily for maintenance. If he wants to build muscle, then he will need an additional 10% calories. This brings Henry's daily calorie intake to 3,300 (3,000 + 10% surplus). Avoid a surplus of over 10% because it increases the chances of fat gain.

Once you have the daily calories, you simply need to determine the number of calories to be obtained from the macros and convert it into grams. So, in Henry's case, his macros breakdown for weight gain and muscle building are as follows.

Protein:

200 x 0.8 = 160 grams of protein

So, the number of calories to be obtained from protein is

160 grams x 4 = 640 calories.

Fats:

200 x 0.35 = 70 grams of fat

So, the number of calories to be obtained from fat is

70 grams x 9 = 630 calories.

Carbohydrates:

Carbs = Total daily calorie consumptions - Total calories from fats and proteins

So, total calories from carbs is

3,300- 640–630 = 2,030 calories.

This is equivalent to 507 grams of carbs (2,030/4)

Key Takeaways

- Before following the macro diet, determine your health or fitness objective.

- Calculation of daily macros is based on the objective you want to attain from the macro diet. This determines your daily calorie requirement too.

- A calorie deficiency or surplus must be maintained for weight loss or gain respectively.

- The daily calorie intake must further be divided as per the macronutrient ratio.

- The ideal macro ratio as per the AMDR is 45–65% calories from carbs, 10–35% from protein, and 20–35% from fats.

- Using the daily calorie and macronutrient breakdown, you can determine the portion of macros you must consume.

Chapter 4: Tracking Your Macros

"A journey of a thousand miles begins with a single step."

Lao Tzu

Follow the Macro Diet

If you have never tracked your macros before, doing this might sound a little overwhelming. However, it is simpler than you think. The most effective means to get started is by making a daily log of everything you eat for a week. This will help determine your average calorie intake. After this, you can start adjusting the macros and increase or decrease the calories, as per your needs. To keep a daily log, maintaining a food journal is a good idea. To make things even easier, these days a variety of apps are available. In the food journal, you must make a note of everything you eat along with the calories present in it. After this, ensure that what you eat is in sync with the desired macros breakdown. Alternatively, an app can do all this for you too!

Set the Target

The first step is to set your target. This means, you need to focus on determining your fitness goal. Unless you know the goal you want to achieve, you cannot calculate the ideal macros. Usually, maintaining a 500 calories deficit per day is ideal for weight and fat loss. On the other hand, increase your consumption by 10% of the maintenance calories for weight gain and muscle building.

As a rule of thumb, reduce your calorie intake by 15–25% for weight loss. On the other hand, increase your calorie intake by 5–15% if you want to gain weight.

Determine the Macro Breakdown

Once you have your target calorie in mind it is time to determine macro requirements depending on your weight. The AMDR recommends that 45–65% of calories must be from carbohydrates, 10–35% from proteins, and 20–35% from fats. Ideally, you will need to consume 0.5–0.8 grams of protein per pound of your body weight. The fat intake on the other hand must be 0.25–0.5 grams per pound of your body weight. The rest of the calories must be from carbohydrates. You were introduced to detailed calculations as well as examples of how to do this in the previous chapter.

Track the Macros and Calories

The simplest way to track your macronutrients and the calories you consume is by maintaining a food journal. These days, a variety of online platforms and applications are also available that can be used for doing the same. Using an online tracker is easier. Some of the popular online trackers to do this are as follows:

- Carb Manager

- LifeSum

- LoseIt!

- MyFitnessPal

- MyMacros+

- Nutritionix Track

Stick to the Diet

Now, all you need to do is track your daily macros. Stick to this diet for at least three weeks to see a positive change. Once you start following the steps mentioned, you will see how easy and sustainable this diet is!

Other Factors

You will need to spend some time and find a macronutrient ratio that works well for your lifestyle. Since there is no optimal ratio for everyone, see what works for you. Ensure that you follow your chosen dietary plan for at least 10 days to see a change. You can opt for a low carb or even a high fat plan and see what works.

You must focus on important lifestyle aspects such as proper sleep, hydration level, stress, and exercise regimen. These are the pillars upon which healthy living rests. even if one of them is compromised your overall sense of well-being reduces. Ensure that you get around seven hours of undisturbed sleep every night. Learn to manage your stress because excess stress makes it difficult to follow a diet. It also increases the likelihood of opting for unhealthy foods. Ensure that you keep your body thoroughly hydrated by drinking at least eight glasses of water daily. You'll need to drink more water if you lead an active lifestyle. Encourage yourself to move your body and do any physical activity for at least 20 minutes daily.

Points to Remember

An important thing you must remember when it comes to the macro diet is the calculations are not absolute by any means. Instead, they provide a general framework or a set of guidelines established based on the average macronutrient ratio. This ratio ensures your body gets its essential nutrients. However, you have complete control to determine the macros you want to consume as per your needs or requirements. As long as you are consuming sufficient food to fulfill the basic AMDR you can maintain your health and fitness levels. The macros ratio, as well as the food you will be consuming, will be the same regardless of whether you want to maintain, again, or lose weight. To obtain the required nourishment, you must consume the same amount of the essential nutrients—proteins and fats. The only difference, based on your goals, will be the amount of carbs you will be consuming.

After going through all the information given in this chapter, you would have realized how important macros are for achieving and maintaining your weight loss and health goals. However, it is rather unfortunate that most have a negative association with the AMDR. This negative association can also be due to the simple fact that a lot of Americans are overweight and have a variety of health problems. Please understand that there is nothing wrong with the guidelines. The only problem is the usual nutrition habits they follow. A majority of individuals are consuming calorie-rich meals instead of nutrient-dense ones. This means they are consuming plenty of simple carbs and unhealthy fats without obtaining the daily dose of complex carbs and healthy proteins and fats.

Following the macro diet is not about fixating on the calories you are consuming. For instance, if your usual diet is rich in processed, pre-packaged, fast, and junk food, your body doesn't get its nutrient requirements. You might be well within the daily calorie consumption but you fall short when it comes to nutrients. For instance, a Big Mac combo meal has around 1,080 calories and a large vanilla shake has 820 calories. A blueberry muffin has around 470 calories and a large Coca-Cola has 290 calories. You can probably eat a couple of these items and still be within your daily calorie requirement. However, your body is not getting healthy macros and this is the leading cause of most health problems associated with the modern lifestyle.

The macro diet is not just about weight loss or weight gain and developing lean muscle. Instead, it is ideal for maintaining your health in the long run as well. Understand that the calorie and macronutrient requirements are based on estimates and must be further adjusted as per your existing level of health, metabolic rate, and other lifestyle factors.

Key Takeaways

- Decide the fitness or health goals you want to achieve by following the macros diet.

- Once you have the daily calorie requirement and macros breakdown.

- Commit to this diet and do not deviate.

- After this, track the foods you eat and make a note of the progress you make.

Chapter 5: Meal Planning

"If you keep good food in your fridge, you will eat good food."

Errick McAdams

Meal planning and prepping are incredible ways to make cooking easy. It not only saves time but helps manage the portion sizes as well. It also encourages the creation and maintenance of a healthier relationship with food. If thinking about what your next meal is has become a source of stress, eliminate it through planning and prepping. Home cooking gives you better control over the quality of ingredients used. Another benefit is it reduces your food bill too. You can obtain all these benefits by making some time for meal planning and preparation.

What more? You do not have to look for any macro diet-friendly recipes or meal plans! This book has all the information you need. In this chapter, you will be introduced to different sample meal plans. Depending on your daily calorie requirement, you can either follow the sample plan or create one that follows your tastes and preferences. The idea is to ensure that you stick to the calorie intake by consuming the desired ratio of macronutrients.

Tips for Meal Planning and Prepping

Developing the perfect meal plan for yourself is incredibly simple. The easiest way to do it is by creating a spreadsheet for the meals you want to eat for an entire week. You don't have to wonder what your next meal will be once you have the meal plan in place.

Doing a little prep over the weekend also makes it easier. To ensure this diet doesn't feel too restrictive, leave a little wiggle room for snacks. You can add or reduce calories from your meal plan based on your requirements. For instance, leaving a buffer of 100–200 calories daily is a good idea. Depending on whether you want to lose or gain weight, the calorie consumption will vary.

Instead of munching on junk food, opt for healthier options such as a protein powder smoothie made with fruits berries, and other natural ingredients, a bowl of fruits, and nuts and seeds. Opting for such healthy snacks also fills any nutritional gaps in your diet. Also, these snacks are incredibly convenient and hardly take any preparation time. Once you go through the sample meal plans discussed in this book, you will get a better idea of how to meet your calorie needs. Further you will find sample 1,500, 2,000, and 2,500 calories meal plans and can adjust them per your individual calorie requirements.

While creating the meal plan, ensure that you take into consideration your usual lifestyle or social commitments. If you are following the 80/20 rule of the macro diet, then you can plan for the 20% calories by taking into consideration your social commitments. This means, you do not have to compromise on your social life for the sake of the diet. It, in turn, makes the diet sustainable and increases your motivation to stick to it.

Always look for recipes that have overlapping ingredients. This makes preparation of the meals incredibly simple. Also, grocery shopping is simplified.

If you want to start meal prepping, then chopping and cooking the staple ingredients is an efficient method. For instance, if you have certain recipes you want to cook in a week, prepare its primary components ahead. If the recipes have overlapping ingredients, then this becomes even simpler. For instance, if most of the recipes have grilled chicken, you can batch cook the chicken over the weekend. The idea of meal planning and prepping is to simplify cooking.

Another efficient means to reduce cooking time is to make the most of your freezer. Any recipe that can be batch-cooked and stored, can be frozen! Soups, curries, stews, and sauces belong to this category. You will simply need to heat the curry, add the protein you have batch cooked, and dinner is ready within no time! A little planning and preparation go a long way!

Before you start meal prepping or planning, ensure that your freezer, pantry, and fridge are stocked with healthy ingredients that you require. Similarly, get rid of all unhealthy foods from your pantry. Out of sight and out of mind, is a great way to go about it. When you have all the required ingredients, cooking also becomes easier.

Sample Meal Plans

Until now you were introduced to different aspects of the macro diet. Now, it is time to make a meal plan for yourself. Meal plan makes it easier to follow the diet. If you usually spend a lot of time wondering what to have for your next meal, then you can stop once you have a meal plan in place. Creating and following a meal plan will ensure you are adhering to your daily macros and calorie count. In this section, you will be introduced to three different types of weekly meal plans based on varying calorie needs. The three categories of calorie requirements are 1,500, 2,000, and 2,500 calories per day. Within these limits, you can consume three meals, a snack, and dessert too! Yes, you read it right! You can have desserts too! All the meal plans can be customized as per your needs and requirements. The meal plans also show the macros breakdown for each of the recipes mentioned along with the recipe numbers. To get started, simply select a meal plan that strikes your fancy or go through the recipes and create one that meets your tastes and preferences

1,500 calories

Day 1

Meal	Recipe Name	Fats (in grams)	Carbs (in grams)	Protein (in grams)	Total calories
Breakfast	#1 Tomato Basil Omelet	21 g	16.5 g	21 g	337.5
Lunch	#22 Lentil Sausage Stew	8 g	34 g	24 g	306
Snack	#70 1 x Coconut Pineapple Shrimp Skewers	2 g	12 g	24 g	165
Dinner	#36 Salsa Spaghetti with Sardines	16 g	43 g	31 g	442
Dessert	#95 Summer Berry Pudding	2.3 g	160.3 g	4.8 g	243
Total		49.3 g	154.4 g	104.8 g	1,493.5

Day 2

Meal	Recipe Name	Fats (in grams)	Carbs (in grams)	Protein (in grams)	Total calories
Breakfast	#4 Breakfast Parfait	4.5 g	66 g	30 g	400.5
Lunch	#17 Spicy Ground Turkey and Green Bean Stir Fry	12 g	11 g	39 g	294
Snack	#72 Crispy Parmesan Garlic Edamame	9 g	8 g	10 g	150
Dinner	#43 Cheeseburger Skillet	16 g	6 g	30 g	325
Side	#77 Healthy Mashed Sweet Potatoes	3 g	24 g	2 g	130
Dessert	#98 Strawberry Nice Cream	0.5 g	22.5 g	1.4 g	191
Total		45 g	137.5 g	112.4 g	1,490.5

Day 3

Meal	Recipe Name	Fats (in grams)	Carbs (in grams)	Protein (in grams)	Total calories
Breakfast	#2 Cranberry Vanilla Oatmeal	15 g	24 g	25 g	368
Lunch	#29 Fish Tacos	4 g	29 g	26 g	254
Snack	#73 Devilled Eggs	4.3	20.1 g	6.6 g	144
Dinner	#34 Salmon and Sweet Potato Grain Bowls	28.9 g	61.1 g	35.5 g	662
Dessert	#89 Birthday Cake Shake	0.5 g	23 g	13.5 g	165
Total		52.7 g	157.2 g	106.6 g	1,593

Day 4

Meal	Recipe Name	Fats (in grams)	Carbs (in grams)	Protein (in grams)	Total calories
Breakfast	#5 Avocado Toast	8 g	28 g	10 g	224
Lunch	#44 Egg Roll Bowl	7.1 g	12.9 g	28.9	233
Snack	#74 Rosemary Roasted Almonds	19.8 g	7.2 g	7.6 g	222
Dinner	#34 Salmon and Sweet Potato Grain Bowl	28.9	61.1 g	35.5 g	662
Dessert	#92 Eggless Chocolate Mousse	1.4 g	22.3 g	7.8 g	127
Total		65.2 g	131.5 g	89.8 g	1,468

Day 5

Meal	Recipe Name	Fats (in grams)	Carbs (in grams)	Protein (in grams)	Total calories
Breakfast	#8 Apple Overnight Oats	13 g	66 g	11 g	405
Lunch	#55 Greek Couscous Salad	25.9 g	31.2 g	9 g	378
Snack	#75 Bruschetta	4.3 g	20.1 g	6.6 g	144
Dinner	#51 Jalapeno Popper Burger	23.5 g	28.6 g	32.8 g	458
Dessert	#88 Brownie	5 g	6 g	14 g	125
Total		71.7 g	151.9 g	73.4 g	1,510

Day 6

Meal	Recipe Name	Fats (in grams)	Carbs (in grams)	Protein (in grams)	Total calories
Breakfast	#10 Breakfast Hash	12 g	26 g	10 g	249
Lunch	#60 Creamy Spinach and Feta Cheese Tortilla Wraps	15 g	28 g	8 g	287
Snack	#69 Baked Spicy Chicken Wings	15 g	1.5 g	9 g	176
Dinner	#25 Sweet Potato and Broccoli Chicken	26 g	47 g	35 g	560
Dessert	#95 Summer Berry Pudding	2.3 g	54.8 g	4.6 g	243
Total		70.3 g	157.3 g	66.6 g	1,515

Day 7

Meal	Recipe Name	Fats (in grams)	Carbs (in grams)	Protein (in grams)	Total calories
Breakfast	#11 Savory Waffles	16 g	44 g	20 g	372
Lunch	#16 Garlic Butter Chicken Meatballs with Cauliflower Rice	24 g	8 g	26 g	342
Snack	#76 Potato Soup	12.1 g	72 g	18.4 g	460
Dinner	#27 Poached Fish in Tomato Basil Sauce	2 g	6 g	32 g	185
Dessert	#91 Pumpkin and Peanut Butter Cup	5 g	20 g	16 g	173
Total		59 g	150 g	112.4 g	1,532

2,000 calories

Day 1

Meal	Recipe Name	Fats (in grams)	Carbs (in grams)	Protein (in grams)	Total calories
Breakfast	#6 Banana and Almond Butter Oatmeal	6 g	66 g	8 g	375
Lunch	#40 Shrimp Pad Thai	16.1 g	64.2 g	15.8 g	462
Snack	#83 Eggplant Parmesan	21 g	16 g	9 g	275
Dinner	#20 Brown Rice Bowl with Turkey	9 g	57 g	42 g	468
Dessert	#96 Grilled Apples with Cheese and Honey	14 g	29.6 g	4.6 g	245
Total		66.1 g	232.8 g	79.4 g	1,825

38

Day 2

Meal	Recipe Name	Fats (in grams)	Carbs (in grams)	Protein (in grams)	Total calories
Breakfast	#12 Green Eggs	20 g	8 g	18 g	298
Lunch	#63 Spicy Tomato and Spinach Pasta	11 g	75 g	24 g	524
Snack	#74 Rosemary Roasted Almonds	19.8 g	7.2 g	7.6 g	222
Dinner	#31 Teriyaki Shrimp Sushi Bowl	30 g	46 g	34 g	584
Dessert	#93 Black Forest Banana Split	11 g	40 g	23 g	377
Total		91.8 g	176.2 g	106.6 g	2,005

Day 3

Meal	Recipe Name	Fats (in grams)	Carbs (in grams)	Protein (in grams)	Total calories
Breakfast	#9 Blueberry Chia Seed Smoothie	4.5 g	46.5 g	22.5 g	309
Lunch	#50 Beef Fajitas	19 g	24 g	35 g	412
Snack	#70 2 x Coconut Pineapple Shrimp Skewers	4 g	24 g	48 g	330
Dinner	#65 Flatbread Pizza	24.9	38.2	38.2	442
Side	#81 Stuffed Delicata Squash	11.2 g	44.5 g	6.5 g	282
Dessert	#90 Gluten-Free Protein Lava Cake	14.8 g	27.5 g	20.1 g	295
Total		78.4 g	204.7 g	170.3 g	2,070

Day 4

Meal	Recipe Name	Fats (in grams)	Carbs (in grams)	Protein (in grams)	Total calories
Breakfast	#7 Strawberry Cheesecake Overnight Oats	5 g	44 g	13 g	271
Lunch	#34 Salmon and Sweet Potato Grain Bowl	28.9	61.1 g	35.5 g	662
Snack	#73 Devilled Eggs	11 g	1 g	7 g	127
Dinner	#54 Orecchiette Pasta	39.1 g	46.2 g	31.2 g	662
Dessert	#94 Marsala Poached Figs Over Ricotta	6.9 g	37.1 g	9 g	228
Total		90.9 g	189.4 g	95.7 g	1,950

Day 5

Meal	Recipe Name	Fats (in grams)	Carbs (in grams)	Protein (in grams)	Total calories
Breakfast	#10 Breakfast hash	12 g	26 g	10 g	249
Lunch	#63 Spicy Tomatoes and Spinach Pasta	11 g	75 g	24 g	524
Snack	#69 Baked Spicy Chicken Wings	15 g	1.5 g	9 g	176
Dinner	#30 Mediterranean Couscous with Tuna and Pepperoni	10 g	52 g	30 g	419
Side	#83 Eggplant Parmesan	21 g	16 g	9 g	275
Dessert	#86 Chocolate Orange Protein Balls	18.3 g	17.25 g	25.3 g	342
Total		87.3 g	187.75 g	107.3 g	1,985

Day 6

Meal	Recipe Name	Fats (in grams)	Carbs (in grams)	Protein (in grams)	Total calories
Breakfast	#3 Sheet Pan Breakfast	34 g	38 g	22 g	546
Lunch	#19 White Bean Turkey Chili	10.1 g	31.9 g	33.2 g	359
Snack	#71 Rainbow Collard Wraps with Peanut Butter Dipping Sauce	35 g	35 g	15 g	476
Dinner	#52 Pork and Bok Choy Stir Fry	6 g	50.9 g	28.6 g	373
Dessert	#96 Grilled Apples with Cheese and Honey	14 g	29.6 g	4.6 g	245
Total		99.1 g	185.4 g	103.4 g	1,999

Day 7

Meal	Recipe Name	Fats (in grams)	Carbs (in grams)	Protein (in grams)	Total calories
Breakfast	#11 Savory Waffles	16 g	44 g	20 g	372
Lunch	#49 Flank Steak Gyros with Quick Pickles	18 g	45 g	33 g	465
Snack	#71 Rainbow Collard Wraps (No Dipping Sauce)	18	25 g	7 g	264
Dinner	#52 Pork and Bok Choy Stir-Fry	16 g	45 g	13 g	375
Side	#81 Stuffed Delicata Squash	11.2 g	44.5	6.5	282
Dessert	#99 Strawberry and Mango Sundae	2.4 g	43.1 g	5.8	206
Total		81.6 g	246.6 g	85.3 g	1,964

2,500 calories

Day 1

Meal	Recipe Name	Fats (in grams)	Carbs (in grams)	Protein (in grams)	Total calories
Breakfast	#2 Cranberry Vanilla Oatmeal	15 g	24 g	25 g	368
Lunch	#4 Brown Rice Bowl with Turkey	9 g	57 g	42 g	468
Snack	#76 Potato Soup	12.1 g	72 g	18.4 g	460
Dinner	#21 Greek Turkey Burgers	15.6 g	26 g	28.4 g	351
Side	#84 Vegetables Stuffed Tomatoes	7 g	23 g	6 g	182
Dessert	#85 Chocolate Chia Pudding	39 g	39 g	8.5 g	517
Total		97.7 g	241 g	128.3 g	2,346

Day 2

Meal	Recipe Name	Fats (in grams)	Carbs (in grams)	Protein (in grams)	Total calories
Breakfast	#4 Breakfast Parfait	4.5 g	66 g	30 g	400.5
Lunch	#46 Lentil Kielbasa Soup	35 g	61 g	34 g	689
Snack	#69 Baked Spicy Chicken Wings	15 g	1.5 g	9 g	176
Dinner	#14 Blackened Chicken Avocado Power Bowl	30 g	28 g	27 g	602
Side	#78 Roasted Vegetables	11 g	23 g	5 g	199
Dessert	#93 Black Forest Banana Split	11 g	40 g	23 g	377
Total		106.5 g	219.5 g	128 g	2,443.5

Day 3

Meal	Recipe Name	Fats (in grams)	Carbs (in grams)	Protein (in grams)	Total calories
Breakfast	#3 Sheet Pan Breakfast	34 g	38 g	22 g	546
Lunch	#40 Shrimp Pad Thai	16.1 g	64.3 g	15.8 g	462
Snack	#73 3x Devilled Eggs	33 g	3 g	21 g	381 (3 x 127)
Dinner	#59 Cauliflower Shawarma Grain Bowl	21 g	64 g	18 g	505
Side	#81 Stuffed Delicata Squash	11.2 g	44.5 g	6.5 g	282
Dessert	#88 Brownie with #87 Chocolate Ice Cream	5 g + 2.2 g (7.2 g)	6 g + 4.5 g (10.5 g)	14 g + 12.75 g (26.75 g)	125 + 180 (305)
Total		122.5 g	224.3 g	110.05 g	2,481

Day 4

Meal	Recipe Name	Fats (in grams)	Carbs (in grams)	Protein (in grams)	Total calories
Breakfast	#6 Banana and Almond Butter Oatmeal	6 g	66 g	8 g	375
Lunch	#54 Orecchiette Pasta with #68 Black Bean Salad	55.1 g (39.1 + 16)	87 g (46.2 g + 40.8)	41.8 g (31.2 g + 10.6)	984 (662 + 322)
Snack	#72 Crispy Parmesan Garlic Edamame	9 g	8 g	10 g	150
Dinner	#63 Spicy Tomatoes and Spinach Pasta	11 g	75 g	24 g	524
Side	#81 Stuffed Delicata Squash	11.2 g	44.5 g	6.5 g	282
Dessert	#94 Marsala Poached Figs Over Ricotta	6.9 g	37.1 g	9 g	228
Total		99.2 g	317.6 g	99.3 g	2,543

Day 5

Meal	Recipe Name	Fats (in grams)	Carbs (in grams)	Protein (in grams)	Total calories
Breakfast	#10 Breakfast Hash #9 Blueberry Chia Seed Smoothie	16.5 g (12 g + 4.5 g)	72.5 g (26 g + 46.5 g)	32.5 g (10 g + 22.5 g)	558 (249 + 309)
Lunch	#39 Shrimp and Avocado Quinoa Bowl #66 Green Goddess Salad with Chickpeas	29.5 g (22 + 7.5)	102.8 g (63 + 39.8)	54.7 g (33 + 21.7)	762 (458 + 304)
Snack	#70 2 x Coconut Pineapple Shrimp Skewers	4 g	24 g	48 g	330 (165 x 2)
Dinner	#48 Steak and Potatoes	20.8	21.5 g	35.1 g	415
Side	#79 Roasted Brussels Sprouts	7.3 g	10 g	2.9 g	104
Dessert	#95 Summer Berry Pudding	2.3 g	54.8 g	4.6 g	243
Total		80.4 g	285.6 g	177.8 g	2,412

Day 6

Meal	Recipe Name	Fats (in grams)	Carbs (in grams)	Protein (in grams)	Total calories
Breakfast	#5 3 x Avocado Toasts	24 g	84 g	30 g	672 (224 x 3)
Lunch	#33 Thai Coconut Curry Shrimp Noodle Bowls	15 g	21 g	15 g	450
Snack	#70 3 x Coconut Pineapple Shrimp Skewers	4 g	24 g	48 g	330 (165 x 2)
Dinner	#65 Flatbread Pizza	24.9 g	38.2 g	17.7 g	442
Side	#82 Sesame Green Beans	16.5 g	8.7 g	3.8 g	196
Dessert	#97 Avocado Ice Cream #88 Chocolate Ice Cream	11.25 g (9 + 2.25)	29.5 g (25 g + 4.5)	15.75 g (3 g + 12.75)	354 (174 + 180)
Total		97.65 g	205.4 g	130.25 g	2,444

Day 7

Meal	Recipe Name	Fats (in grams)	Carbs (in grams)	Protein (in grams)	Total calories
Breakfast	#11 Savory Waffles	16 g	44 g	20 g	372
Lunch	#36 Salsa Spaghetti with Sardines	16 g	43 g	31 g	442
Snack	#76 Potato Soup	12.1 g	72 g	18.4 g	460
Dinner	#49 Flank Steak Gyros with Quick Pickles #67 Spiced Cauliflower and Chickpea Salad	27.4 g (18 + 9.4)	77.6 g (45 + 32.6)	43.6 g (33 + 10.6)	706 (465 + 241)
Dessert	#86 Chocolate Orange Protein Balls #89 Birthday Cake Shake	18.8 g (18.3 + 0.5)	40.25 g (17.25 + 23)	38.8 g (25.3 + 13.5)	507 (342 + 165)
Total		90.3 g	276.85 g	151.8 g	2,487

Chapter 6: FAQs About the

Macros Diet

"Your diet is a bank account. Good food choices are good investments."

Bethenny Frankel

In the chapters until now, you were introduced to different aspects of the macro diet. In this chapter, the most common questions and queries about the macro diet are answered.

Can I Eat Pizza and Lose Weight?

It's been repeatedly mentioned that you do not have to worry too much about what you are eating as long as you stick to the macronutrient intake. It is not a free pass to eat whatever you want and still expect weight loss benefits. It's not just about sticking to your daily calorie or macronutrient intake. Instead, you must make conscious and healthy food choices. It can be quite tempting to think that you can start eating pizza daily to lose weight on this diet. After all, you are sticking to the macronutrient intake! Unfortunately, this is not how it works. The quality of calories along with the food you eat matters a lot.

It is not a reason to give up on the notion of sensible eating. It is not a pro-junk food diet. For instance, calories are present in a piece of cake as well as a bowl of salad. That said, only one of them is healthy. If you are constantly eating unhealthy foods, you are not only depriving your body of the nourishment it needs but are increasing empty calorie consumption. This will ultimately result in weight gain. If you can occasionally indulge in your guilty pleasures but ensure it is occasional and not the norm.

Is Alcohol a Carbohydrate and How Does It Affect My Diet?

Drinking alcohol makes it harder to lose weight and there is no way around it. There are different reasons and the most important one is that alcohol is rich in calories. This coupled with any mixers simply increases your calorie consumption. These are empty calories and do not offer any nutrients whatsoever. Drinking alcohol reduces your inhibitions which makes it easier to overindulge and eat unhealthy foods. It also interferes with your body's ability to burn fat.

If you are following the macro diet to improve your health or achieve and maintain your weight loss benefits, then staying away from alcohol is a good idea. You might not have realized but even a seemingly small glass of white wine has 121 calories. A regular beer of 12 ounces has 153 calories whereas 1.5 oz of whiskey, rum, vodka, and tequila has 97 calories in it. So, avoiding these calories is a better idea.

What If I Don't Have the Time to Cook Daily?

We all lead hectic lives these days. This means, most of us don't have time to cook daily. Home-cooked meals are the best means to ensure your body gets nutrients. It's also needed to ensure you consume healthy and wholesome meals. However, this might not be an option for everyone. In such instances, the urge to eat out or order taken increases. It also increases the dependence on processed and pre-packaged foods. To ensure you do not fall into this trap, create a weekly meal plan. Once the meal plan is in place, you can do the required prep over the weekend. Spending as little as 2–3 hours over the weekend makes it easier to cook wholesome meals during the week.

Select the recipes you like from this book or even opt for one of the sample meal plans. shop for the required groceries and stock your pantry. You can batch cook a specific sauce or even a recipe and store it. Similarly, vegetables and proteins can be portioned as per your daily requirements. Some recipes can be cooked and frozen. Then all you need to do is reheat it and a meal is ready.

Do I Need Any Supplements?

The macro diet focuses on your consumption of macronutrients. That said, micronutrients are equally important. If you are worried about not meeting your body's daily nutritional needs then consult your healthcare provider and use a nutrient supplement. That said, if you are consuming healthy and wholesome ingredients, this is not something you should even have to worry about. Do not add any supplements to your diet without consulting a professional.

Do I Need to Exercise Regularly?

The diet you follow plays a significant role in your overall health and well-being. You should also focus on your level of physical activity if you want to achieve and maintain your health and fitness goals. Exercising regularly is needed for improving your physical and mental health. You don't have to spend hours together at the gym to exercise. Instead, playing a sport or exercising for about 30 minutes daily also does the trick. Find an activity that you like and engage in that regularly.

How Do I Balance My Macros While Eating Out?

You do not have to worry about giving up on the diet when you are eating out. You can plan your day such that it does not clash with your social calendar. Following the 80/20 rule ensures that at least 80% of your daily calories are from nutrient-dense ingredients. The rest can be used for guilty pleasures. Why don't you consider saving 20% of your daily calories when you are eating out? This makes it easy.

Another option at your disposal is to be mindful of the food choices you make even when eating out. These days, restaurants offer a variety of healthy food options. Whether it is a salad, appetizer, or even an entrée, opt for something that caters to your macro requirements.

Key Takeaways

- The macro diet is easy, simple and sustainable. It requires commitment, consistency, and patience.

- Following this diet is not an excuse to binge on unhealthy foods. Instead, it's about making conscious food choices.

- Avoid alcohol, sugar-laden beverages, and other junk food if you want to optimize the benefits offered by this diet.

- With a little careful consideration, planning, and preparation, following the diet is perfectly easy and doable.

Chapter 7: Recipes

Understanding the nutritional profile of the food you eat makes it easier to ensure you are hitting your daily macros goals while adhering to the calorie limit. You needn't look any further for macro diet-friendly recipes because this chapter contains a variety of recipes. All the recipes are divided into different categories for your convenience. While selecting recipes for your macros diet meal plan, don't forget about your daily calorie targets. If you need additional calories or carbs, add a serving of a side dish, salad, or a snack

All the recipes are for one serving. The nutritional values are for one serving.

A quick note before we start with recipes.

To keep our books at a reasonable price for you, we print in black & white.

To get recipe images in full color scan with your camera

Breakfast and Brunch Recipes

Discover easy-to-cook and nutritious breakfast and brunch recipes to ensure that your day is off to a good start! Fill up on the essential macros to ensure your body has sufficient energy to get through your day.

1. Tomato Basil Omelet

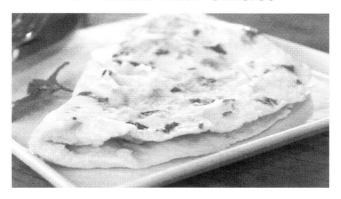

Nutritional values:

- Calories: 337.5
- Fat: 21 g
- Carbohydrate: 16.5 g
- Protein: 21 g

Ingredients:

- 3 eggs
- 1 ½ teaspoons olive oil
- 6 large basil leaves, thinly sliced + extra to serve
- Pine nuts to serve (optional)
- 3 tablespoons whole milk
- Salt and pepper to taste
- 4 cherry tomatoes, halved

Directions:

1. Whisk together eggs, milk, salt, and pepper in a bowl with a fork.
2. Pour oil into a medium pan and let it heat over medium heat.
3. Swirl the pan to spread the oil. Add egg mixture into the pan and tilt the pan to spread the egg all around the pan.
4. Scatter tomatoes and basil on one half of the omelet. Sprinkle salt and pepper to taste. When the eggs are set, loosen the omelet by sliding a spatula below the omelet
5. Fold the other half of the omelet over the filling.
6. Press lightly. Slide the omelet onto a plate and serve garnished with pine nuts and basil.
7. You can replace the tomatoes with any other vegetable of your choice. You can replace the pine nuts with any other nuts of your choice. Of course the nutritional value will change.

2. Cranberry Vanilla Oatmeal

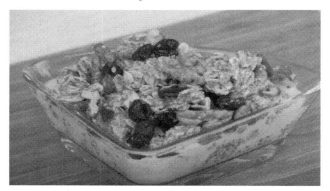

Nutritional values:

- Calories: 368

- Fat: 15 g

- Carbohydrate: 24 g

- Protein: 25 g

Ingredients:

- 1 cup almond milk, unsweetened

- 1 ½ tablespoons dried cranberries

- ¼ teaspoon ground cinnamon

- 1 teaspoon light brown sugar (optional)

- ½ cup oatmeal

- ½ teaspoon vanilla extract

- 1 tablespoon chopped walnuts

Directions:

1. Combine oatmeal, almond milk, vanilla, cranberries, and cinnamon in a small saucepan.

2. Place the saucepan over low heat and cook until well combined. Add brown sugar if using. The nutritional value of brown sugar is not included.

3. Serve in a bowl garnished with walnuts and some cranberries.

3. Sheet Pan Breakfast

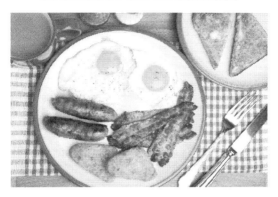

Nutritional values:

- Calories: 546
- Fat: 34 g
- Carbohydrate: 38 g
- Protein: 22 g

Ingredients:

- 2 slices bacon
- 2 eggs
- ¼ cup shredded cheddar cheese
- 2 breakfast sausage links
- Pepper to taste
- 3.75 ounces frozen hash brown
- Salt to taste

Directions:

1. Start off by preheating your oven to 375 °F.
2. Take a baking sheet and spray it with some cooking spray.
3. Place sausages and hash browns on the baking sheet.
4. Place the baking sheet in the oven and set the timer for 25 minutes.
5. After baking for 10 minutes, take out the baking sheet and place bacon on the baking sheet. Put the baking sheet back in the oven and continue cooking for the remaining 15 minutes.
6. Take out the baking sheet and break the eggs on the baking sheet. Season with salt and pepper. Sprinkle salt and pepper on the hash browns as well.
7. Set the timer for 12 minutes and place the baking sheet back in the oven.
8. Scatter cheese over the ingredients on the baking sheet after about 8–9 minutes of baking.
9. Serve hot.

4. Breakfast Parfait

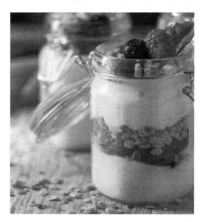

Nutritional values:

- Calories: 400.5

- Fat: 4.5 g

- Carbohydrate: 66 g

- Protein: 30 g

Ingredients:

- 9 ounces Greek yogurt

- 6 tablespoons granola

- ¾ cup berries of your choice

- ¾ teaspoon honey

Directions:

1. Take a Mason's jar or a parfait glass. Place some yogurt at the bottom of the glass. Place some berries over the granola followed by some yogurt.

2. Repeat this layering until all the berries, granola and yogurt is used up.

3. Drizzle honey on top and serve.

5. Avocado Toast

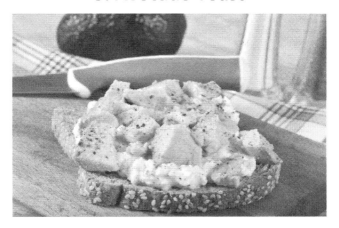

Nutritional values:

- Calories: 224
- Fat: 8 g
- Carbohydrate: 28 g
- Protein: 10 g

Ingredients:

- ¼ medium ripe avocado, peeled, pitted, mashed
- ¼ teaspoon lime juice or to taste
- Sea salt to taste
- Red chili flakes to taste
- Hot sauce to taste (optional)
- 1.3 ounces low-fat (1%) cottage cheese
- 1 slice whole-grain bread
- Pepper to taste

Directions:

1. Combine cottage cheese and avocado in a bowl. Mash them up using a fork.

2. Add lime juice, pepper, and salt and stir.

3. Toast the slice of bread to the desired doneness. Spread the avocado-cheese mixture over the toast.

4. Sprinkle red chili flakes on top. Drizzle with hot sauce on top if using and serve.

5. You can have 2 or 3 avocado toasts to meet up with your calorie requirements.

6. Banana and Almond Butter Oatmeal

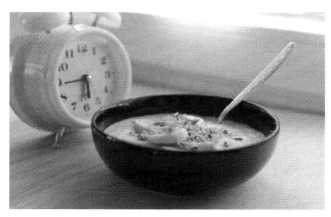

Nutritional values:

- Calories: 375

- Fat: 6 g

- Carbohydrate: 66 g

- Protein: 8 g

Ingredients:

- 1 cup unsweetened almond milk

- ½ banana, sliced

- 1 teaspoon honey (optional)

- ½ cup steel cut or old fashioned oats

- 1 tablespoon almond butter

Directions:

1. Add oats and almond milk into a saucepan. Place the saucepan over low heat and cook until nearly dry.

2. Stir in half the banana slices and almond butter and cook until you get the desired consistency.

3. Turn off the heat. Spoon the oatmeal into a bowl. Top with honey and remaining banana slices and serve. Nutritional value of honey is not included. You can also add 1 or ½ scoop of whey protein if you need extra protein to hit your macros.

7. Strawberry Cheesecake Overnight Oats

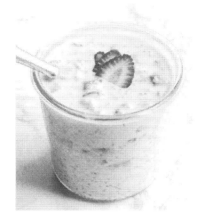

Nutritional values:

- Calories: 271
- Fat: 5 g
- Carbohydrate: 44 g
- Protein: 13 g

Ingredients:

- ½ cup rolled oats
- ½ tablespoon chia seeds
- ½ cup diced strawberries
- A wee bit salt
- 4 tablespoons nonfat, plain Greek yogurt
- ½ teaspoon vanilla extract
- 6 tablespoons unsweetened almond milk or milk of your choice
- ½ tablespoon honey
- Crushed Graham crackers to serve (optional)
- Strawberry jam to serve (optional)

Directions:

1. Add strawberries, Greek yogurt, and almond milk into a blender and blend until smooth.
2. Pour into a bowl. Add honey and stir. Add rolled oats, salt, vanilla extract, and chia seeds and stir.
3. Cover the bowl and chill for 6–8 hours.
4. Place the graham crackers and strawberry jam on top and serve. The nutritional value of graham crackers and strawberry jam are not included.

8. Apple Overnight Oats

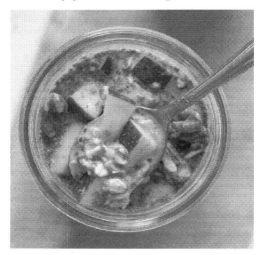

Nutritional values:

- Calories: 405

- Fat: 13 g

- Carbohydrate: 66 g

- Protein: 11 g

Ingredients:

- ½ apple, thinly sliced

- 1 tablespoon almond butter

- ½ teaspoon lemon juice

- ½ cup rolled oats or steel cut oats

- 1 tablespoon raisins

- 1 tablespoon brown sugar

- ¼ teaspoon ground cinnamon

- A wee bit salt

- ¼ cup milk of your choice

Directions:

1. Combine almond butter, brown sugar, apple, cinnamon, salt, and lemon juice into a small saucepan.

2. Place the saucepan over low heat and cook until the apples are soft. Turn off the heat.

3. Place oats in a bowl or jar. Place the apple mixture over the oats. Drizzle milk on top. Scatter raisins. Stir if desired. Keep the bowl covered and chill for 6–8 hours.

4. You can serve this cold or warm. You can warm it in a microwave.

9. Blueberry Chia Seed Smoothie

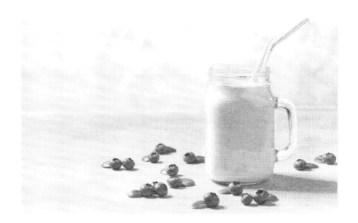

Nutritional values:

- Calories: 309
- Fat: 4.5 g
- Carbohydrate: 46.5 g
- Protein: 22.5 g

Ingredients:

- ¾ cup blueberries
- ¾ banana, sliced
- ¾ cup cubed cantaloupe
- ¾ tablespoon chia seeds
- 6 tablespoons milk (optional)
- ¾ cup Greek yogurt
- ¾ tablespoon honey (optional)

Directions:

1. Blend together blueberries, cantaloupe, Greek yogurt, and banana in a blender until very smooth.

2. Add milk or water if the smoothie is very thick. Add chia seeds and honey if using and blend until smooth.

3. Pour smoothie into a glass. Let the smoothie rest for 20 minutes in the refrigerator. The chia seeds will swell up.

4. Serve. The nutritional value of optional ingredients is not included.

10. Breakfast Hash

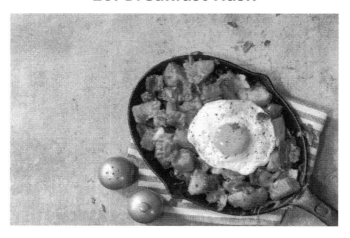

Nutritional values:

- Calories: 249
- Fat: 12 g
- Carbohydrate: 26 g
- Protein: 10 g

Ingredients:

- 1 egg
- ½ medium onion, diced
- ½ teaspoon paprika
- 1 tablespoon olive oil
- 2 small cloves garlic, sliced
- ½ large potato, cubed
- 1 ½ rashers bacon (optional)
- ½ tablespoon chopped fresh parsley
- ½ red bell pepper, diced
- Chopped avocado to serve
- Salt to taste
- Pepper to taste

Directions:

1. Pour oil into a skillet and let it heat over medium heat. When oil is hot, add potatoes and cook for a few minutes until slightly tender. Stir occasionally.

2. Stir in garlic, bell pepper, bacon, and onion. Turn down the heat to low heat and cook for about 4 to 5 minutes.

3. Add salt, pepper, and paprika and stir. Cover the pan and cook until the potatoes are fork tender.

4. Make a cavity in the center of the hash. Crack the egg into the cavity. Season the egg with salt and pepper.

5. Once the egg is cooked to your preference, turn off the heat.

6. Transfer hash and egg onto a plate. Garnish with parsley and serve topped with avocado. You can serve the hash with bread if desired. The nutritional values of bacon and bread are not included.

11. Savory Waffles

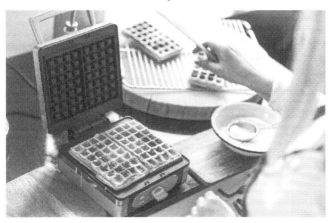

Nutritional values:

- Calories: 372
- Fat: 16 g
- Carbohydrate: 44 g
- Protein: 20 g

Ingredients:

- 1 medium carrot, peeled, grated
- ⅓ cup grated cheese
- ½ spring onion, finely chopped
- 1 egg, lightly beaten
- ½ small sweet potato, peeled, grated
- 2 ⅔ tablespoons whole-meal flour
- 1 teaspoon chopped fresh parsley
- Salt and pepper to taste

Directions:

1. Combine carrot, cheese, sweet potato, spring onion, salt, pepper, and parsley in a bowl. Let it sit for 5 to 8 minutes.
2. Add whole meal flour and stir. Add the beaten egg and mix well.
3. Set up your waffle maker and preheat it following the manufacturer's instructions.
4. You can make either 2 regular size waffles or 4 mini waffles.
5. Spray the waffle iron with cooking spray. Scoop out ¼ of the batter and pour into the waffle maker. Spread the batter if it is very thick.
6. Close the lid and cook the waffle for about 5 minutes or the way you prefer it cooked.
7. Take out the waffle and keep it on a wire rack.
8. Make the remaining waffles in a similar manner.
9. Serve.

12. Green Eggs

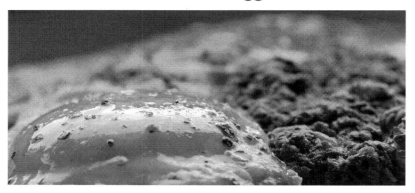

Nutritional values:

- Calories: 298
- Fat: 20 g
- Carbohydrate: 8 g
- Protein: 18 g

Ingredients:

- 1 ½ teaspoons cooking oil
- 1 clove garlic, peeled, sliced
- ¼ teaspoon fennel seeds
- 1 large egg
- Lemon juice to drizzle
- 1 leek, sliced
- ¼ teaspoon coriander seeds
- Chili flakes to taste + extra to garnish
- 1 tablespoon Greek yogurt
- 3.5 ounces spinach
- Salt to taste

Directions:

1. Pour half the oil into a pan and let it heat over medium heat.
2. When oil is hot, add leeks and a bit of salt and cook until tender.
3. Stir in garlic, fennel seeds, and coriander seeds. Cook for a few seconds, until you get a nice aroma.
4. Stir in chili flakes and spinach. Reduce the heat and cook until spinach wilts.
5. Move the spinach mixture to one side of the pan. Add remaining oil in the center of the pan.
6. When the oil is hot, crack the egg over the oil and cook the eggs, sunny side up or as per your preference.
7. Turn off the heat.
8. Drizzle yogurt over the spinach mixture and stir. Transfer the greens onto a serving plate. Add salt and pepper to taste.
9. Place egg over the greens. Sprinkle salt, chili flakes, and pepper over the egg. Drizzle some lemon juice on top and serve.

Poultry Recipes

13. Chicken Salad

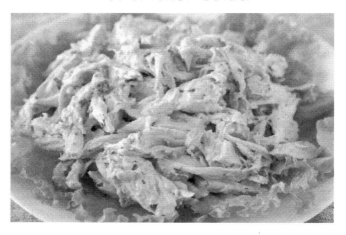

Nutritional values:

- Calories: 779
- Fat: 63.1 g
- Carbohydrate: 8.4 g
- Protein: 44.3 g

Ingredients:

- ¼ cup blanched, slivered almonds
- 1–2 teaspoons fresh lemon juice
- 1 cup cooked, cubed chicken meat
- 4 tablespoons mayonnaise
- Freshly cracked pepper to taste
- ½ stalk celery, chopped
- Sea salt to taste
- 1 teaspoon chopped chives (optional)

Directions:

1. Place chicken pieces in a bowl. Add remaining ingredients and chives if using. Mix well. Taste the salad and add salt if required.

2. You can serve it just like it is prepared or place it on lettuce leaves or use it as a filling for sandwiches or wraps and serve. The nutritional values of the bread or wraps are not included.

14. Blackened Chicken Avocado Power Bowl

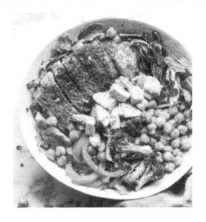

Nutritional values:

- Calories: 602
- Fat: 30 g
- Carbohydrate: 28 g
- Protein: 57 g

Ingredients:

- ½ teaspoon chili powder or to taste
- ¼ teaspoon onion powder
- 1/8 teaspoon garlic powder
- ½ teaspoon paprika
- Pepper to taste
- ¼ teaspoon ground cumin
- ¼ teaspoon Italian seasoning
- Salt to taste
- 1 regular size (around 4 oz) chicken breast, cut into thin slices
- ½ cup broccoli florets
- ¼ yellow bell pepper, sliced
- ¼ red bell pepper, sliced
- 1 tablespoon olive oil, divided
- ¼ can (from a 15 ounces can) chickpeas, drained, rinsed
- ¼ avocado, peeled, pitted, chopped
- ¼ cup chopped red cabbage

Directions:

1. Firstly you have to rub the chicken with spices. For this, combine chili powder, onion powder, garlic powder, salt, paprika, cumin, Italian seasoning, and pepper in a bowl. Sprinkle a little of the spice mixture over the chicken and rub it into it.

2. Pour 1/3 of the oil into a skillet and place the skillet over medium-high heat. When oil is hot, place chicken in the pan and cook for a couple of minutes on each side.

3. The next step is to roast the vegetables. Preheat your oven to 425 °F.

4. Place broccoli, bell peppers and chickpeas on a baking sheet. Pour remaining oil over the vegetables and mix well. Sprinkle salt, pepper, and a little of the spice mixture. Toss well. Spread it evenly.

5. Put the baking sheet in the oven and set the timer for 15 minutes or until the vegetables are tender.

6. To serve: Place the roasted vegetables, avocado and red cabbage in the bowl. Top with chicken pieces and serve.

PS: If you feel the portion size is too much, you can eat it over two meals during the day or you can serve this for 2 people or prepare 1/2 portion at once.

15. Buffalo Chicken

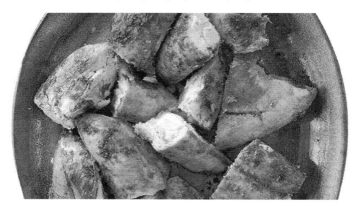

Nutritional values:

- Calories: 320
- Fat: 13 g
- Carbohydrate: 25 g
- Protein: 24 g

Ingredients:

- 4 ounces boneless chicken breast or thighs
- ¾ tablespoon ghee or coconut oil or butter
- ¼ teaspoon garlic powder
- 2 tablespoons hot pepper sauce
- ¾ tablespoon coconut aminos
- 1/8 teaspoon cayenne pepper or to taste (optional)

To serve:

- Ranch dressing (optional)
- 1 small sweet potato (about 7 ounces raw), baked

Directions:

1. This recipe will best get cooked in a slow cooker or an instant pot. So go ahead and use it if you have one. I am going to tell you how to cook it without the slow cooker or an instant pot, on your stovetop.

2. Add hot sauce, garlic powder, coconut aminos, ghee, and cayenne pepper in a small saucepan. Place the saucepan over low heat. Stir until the ghee melts. Turn off the heat.

3. Place a nonstick pan over medium heat. Place chicken in the pan and cook until the underside is golden brown or the way you prefer it to be cooked. Turn the chicken over and cover the pan. Cook the other side until golden brown and the chicken is well cooked inside.

4. Take out the chicken from the pan and place it on your cutting board. After resting the chicken for 5 minutes, cut into slices.

5. Add chicken into the sauce mixture. Mix well and serve with ranch dressing if using and sweet potato. The nutritional value of ranch dressing is not included.

16. Garlic Butter Chicken Meatballs with Cauliflower Rice

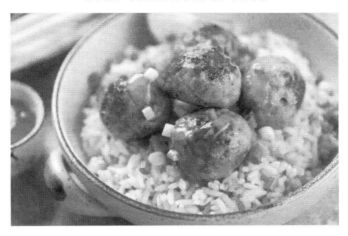

Nutritional values:

- Calories: 342

- Fat: 24 g

- Carbohydrate: 8 g

- Protein: 26 g

Ingredients:

- 4 ounces ground chicken or turkey

- 1 clove garlic, grated

- 1 small clove garlic, minced

- 1/8 teaspoon crushed red pepper flakes (optional)

- 2 tablespoons chicken stock

- 2 tablespoons chopped fresh parsley or cilantro, divided

- ½–1 teaspoon hot sauce

- 2 tablespoons shredded cheese of your preference

- ¼ teaspoon Italian seasoning

- ¼ teaspoon crumbled bouillon cube (optional)

- Salt to taste

- 1 ½ teaspoons butter, divided

- ¼ medium head cauliflower, grated to rice like texture

- Freshly cracked pepper to taste

Directions:

1. Place cauliflower rice in a microwave safe bowl. Sprinkle some water over the rice and cover it with a lid. Cook on high for about 2 minutes. Check if the cauliflower

rice is cooked. If not, cook for a few more seconds.

2. To make meatballs: Add ground chicken, grated garlic, bouillon cube, half the parsley, cheese, Italian seasoning, red pepper flakes, and cracked pepper into a bowl and mix it up using your hands. Make small meatballs of the mixture and keep them on a plate.

3. Add half the butter into a skillet and let it melt over medium-low heat. Add meatballs and cook until brown all over and well-cooked inside. As the meatballs are cooking, drizzle the cooked juices over the meatballs.

4. Transfer the meatballs onto a plate and keep it aside.

5. Add remaining butter into the skillet. When butter melts, add stock, lemon juice, minced garlic, hot sauce, red pepper flakes, and remaining parsley and mix well. Cook for a couple of minutes. Add salt and pepper to taste and turn off the heat.

6. To serve: Place cauliflower rice in a bowl. Place meatballs over the cauliflower rice. Pour the sauce over the meatballs and cauliflower rice and serve. You can also use regular rice instead of cauliflower rice. The nutritional values will change as cauliflower rice is a healthier option.

7. You can make this ahead of time and place the chicken, rice, and sauce in meal prep containers in the refrigerator.

8. Reheat in a microwave and serve.

17. Spicy Ground Turkey and Green Bean Stir—Fry

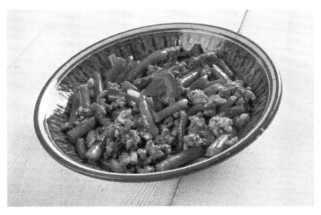

Nutritional values:

- Calories: 294
- Fat: 12 g
- Carbohydrate: 11 g
- Protein: 39 g

Ingredients:

- 4 ounces green beans
- ¾ teaspoon sesame oil
- ½ tablespoon minced ginger
- 1 tablespoon low-sodium soy sauce
- ½ teaspoon sambal oelek (Asian chili garlic paste) or Sriracha
- 2 teaspoons coconut oil or vegetable oil
- 1 small clove garlic, minced
- 1/3 pound 99% lean ground turkey
- ½ tablespoon rice vinegar

Directions:

1. Set the oven to broil mode and preheat the oven. Drizzle 1 teaspoon vegetable oil over the green beans and place them on a sheet of foil. Wrap it up and place it on a baking sheet.

2. Set the timer for 6–8 minutes or until cooked and slightly charred.

3. Pour remaining vegetable oil and sesame oil into a pan and place the pan over medium-high heat. When oil is hot, add garlic, turkey, and ginger and cook until the meat is brown. As you stir, break the meat.

4. Stir in the broiled green beans, vinegar, soy sauce, and sambal oelek. Once it is mixed well, taste a bit of it and add more soy sauce if necessary.

5. Serve

18. Pita Pepperoni Pizza

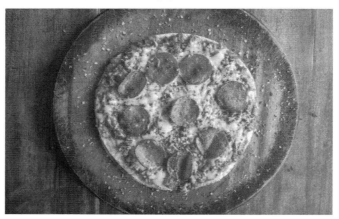

Nutritional values:

- Calories: 237.5
- Fat: 11.5 g
- Carbohydrate: 17 g
- Protein: 23 g

Ingredients:

- 1 whole wheat pita bread
- ¼ cup shredded mozzarella cheese
- ¼ cup low-fat ricotta cheese
- Red pepper flakes to taste
- 8 slices (65% less fat) turkey pepperoni
- ¼ cup Italian herb pasta sauce
- ½ tablespoon grated parmesan cheese

Directions:

1. Start off by preheating your oven to 350 °F.

2. Place the rack in the center of the oven. Place the pita on the rack and bake for 3 minutes or until slightly crisp. Make sure it does not brown.

3. Spread tomato sauce over the pita. Place pepperoni slices. Scatter mozzarella cheese over the pepperoni slices. Place pieces of ricotta all over.

4. Put the pita on a baking sheet and place the baking sheet in the oven. Bake for a few more minutes until the cheese melts and the pita is slightly brown around the edges.

5. Sprinkle parmesan cheese on top. Sprinkle red pepper on top and serve.

19. White Bean Turkey Chili

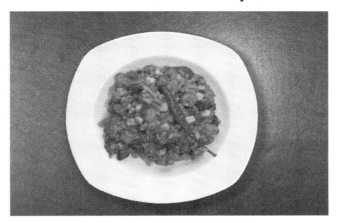

Nutritional values:

- Calories: 359
- Fat: 10.1 g
- Carbohydrate: 31.9 g
- Protein: 33.2 g

Ingredients:

- ¾ teaspoon extra-virgin olive oil
- 1 clove garlic, chopped
- 4 ounces 98% lean ground turkey
- ¼ can (from a 9.2 ounces can) cannellini beans or white kidney beans, rinsed, drained
- ¾ teaspoon tomato paste
- ¼ teaspoon reduced-sodium chicken base
- ¼ teaspoon black pepper
- 1/8 teaspoon garlic powder
- 1/8 teaspoon chili powder
- ¼ teaspoon red pepper flakes
- A pinch ground oregano
- ½ small onion, chopped
- ¼ medium orange bell pepper, diced
- ¼ jalapeño pepper, diced
- ½ can (from a 14 ounces can) petite diced tomatoes in tomato juice
- ½ can (from a 5.6 ounces can) sweet corn
- ¼ cup water, salt to taste

Directions:

1. Pour oil into a heavy pot and place it over medium heat. Once the oil is hot, add onion, bell pepper, and garlic and cook until slightly soft. Stir regularly.

2. Stir in ground turkey. As you stir, break the meat into smaller pieces. Cook until the meat is not pink anymore.

3. Stir in beans, jalapeño, tomato paste, tomatoes, corn, water, chicken base, salt, and spices and mix well.

4. Close the pot and let it simmer for 7–8 minutes. Uncover and mix well.

5. Turn down the heat to low heat and simmer for 10 minutes, making sure to stir every couple of minutes.

6. Serve hot.

20. Brown Rice Bowl with Turkey

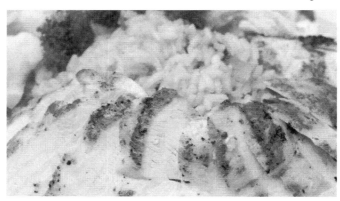

Nutritional values:

- Calories: 468
- Fat: 9 g
- Carbohydrate: 57 g
- Protein: 42 g

Ingredients:

- 1/3 cup short grain brown rice
- ¾ cup low-sodium chicken broth, divided
- ¾ teaspoon olive oil
- ¾ teaspoon low-sodium soy sauce, divided
- ¼ bunch scallions, chopped
- ¾ teaspoon sesame seeds, toasted (optional)
- Kosher salt to taste
- ½ pound bone-in turkey breast
- Freshly ground pepper to taste
- 1 cup baby spinach
- ¾ teaspoon sesame oil

Directions:

1. To cook rice. Place a medium size saucepan over medium heat. Add rice, ½ cup broth, salt to taste and ¼ cup water. Cover with a lid.
2. When the liquid in the saucepan starts boiling, turn down the heat. Simmer until the rice is tender. Add more water if required.
3. Set the temperature of your oven to 425 °F and preheat the oven.
4. Prepare a baking sheet by lining it with foil. Spray with cooking spray.
5. Sprinkle salt and pepper over the turkey and keep it on the baking sheet. Brush half the soy sauce over the turkey.
6. Place the baking sheet in the oven and set the timer for 30–40 minutes or until cooked through. Turn the turkey breast over after about 20 minutes of roasting. The internal temperature of the well-cooked turkey should show 165 °F on a meat thermometer.
7. Remove the turkey from the oven and place it on your cutting board. Cover loosely with foil. Let it sit for 5 minutes. Cut the turkey into thin slices.
8. Add scallions, spinach and remaining soy sauce into the rice. Heat up the remaining broth and pour into the rice. Mix well.
9. Serve rice in a bowl. Top with turkey slices. Trickle sesame oil and scatter sesame seeds on top and serve.

21. Greek Turkey Burgers

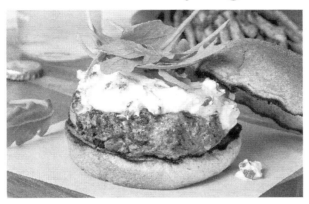

Nutritional values:
- Calories: 351
- Fat: 15.6 g
- Carbohydrate: 26 g
- Protein: 28.4 g

Ingredients:

For the burger:
- 4 ounces ground turkey breast
- 1 teaspoon chopped fresh oregano
- 1/8 teaspoon salt or to taste
- ¾ tablespoon extra-virgin olive oil
- ¼ teaspoon crushed red pepper
- 1 clove garlic, peeled, grated

To serve:
- 1/8 cup thinly sliced onion
- 1/8 cup crumbled feta cheese
- ¼ cup baby spinach leaves
- ¾ teaspoon red wine vinegar or any vinegar
- 1 whole-wheat burger bun, split into two

Directions:
1. Place turkey, oregano, oil, salt, red pepper, and garlic in a bowl and mix using your hand.
2. Shape into a patty of about ½ inch thickness.
3. Place a nonstick pan over medium heat. Spray the pan with cooking spray. Place the burger in the pan and cook until brown on both the sides and cooked through inside. The internal temperature of the cooked turkey burger should show 155 °F on a meat thermometer.
4. To serve: Combine vinegar, onion, and spinach in a bowl.
5. Toast the burger bun to the desired doneness on one side or both sides, as per your preference.
6. Spread 1 tablespoon feta on the cut part of each burger half.
7. Lay the burger on the bottom half of the bun. Spread spinach mixture over the burger. Cover with the top half of the bun and serve.

22. Lentil Sausage Stew

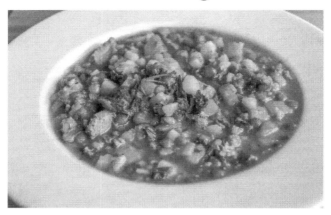

Nutritional values:

- Calories: 306
- Fat: 8 g
- Carbohydrate: 34 g
- Protein: 24 g

Ingredients:

- ½ teaspoon olive oil
- ¼ green bell pepper, chopped
- 1 clove garlic, minced
- ¾ cup chicken broth
- ¼ teaspoon fennel seeds
- ¼ cup chopped onions
- 4 ounces Italian style turkey sausage crumbled
- ½ cup dry lentils, rinsed
- ¼ can (from a 14.1 ounces can) low-sodium tomatoes with its juice
- ¼ teaspoon dried Italian seasoning
- Black pepper to taste
- Salt to taste

Directions:

1. If you have time on hand, soak the lentils for about an hour. Pour oil into a skillet and let it heat over medium heat. When the oil is hot, add onion and bell pepper and sauté until tender.

2. Add sausage and garlic and sauté until it is not pink any more. Break the meat as you stir.

3. Add lentils, broth, tomatoes with its juice, Italian seasoning, fennel seeds, and pepper.

4. Turn down the heat. Cook covered until the lentils are soft.

5. Add salt and simmer for 5 minutes. If at any time there is no liquid in the pan, Add more broth or water.

6. Taste and adjust the seasoning if necessary.

7. Ladle into a bowl and serve with a grain of your choice like quinoa, brown rice etc., the nutritional value of the grain is not included.

23. Orzo Chicken Salad with Avocado Lime Dressing

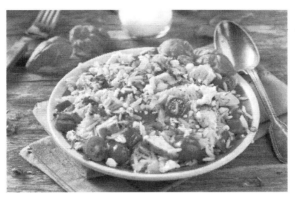

Nutritional values:

- Calories: 321
- Fat: 10 g
- Carbohydrate: 30 g
- Protein: 30 g

Ingredients:

For the dressing:

- ¼ small avocado, peeled, pitted, chopped
- 1/8 teaspoon grated lime zest
- 1 clove garlic, peeled, minced
- Salt to taste
- 1–2 tablespoons water
- 1–2 tablespoons lemon juice
- Crushed red pepper flakes to taste

For salad:

- 3 tablespoons dried whole-wheat orzo pasta
- ½ cup skinless, boneless, chopped, cooked chicken breast
- 1 tablespoon chopped fresh cilantro
- ¼ cup fresh or frozen corn kernels
- ¼ cup halved grape tomatoes
- 1/8 cup crumbled low-fat feta cheese

Directions:

1. To make dressing: Add avocado, lime zest, garlic, water, red pepper flakes, lemon juice, and salt into a blender and blend until smooth. Pour into a bowl. Cover and set aside in the refrigerator for a couple of hours to chill.

2. To make salad: Cook the orzo following the instructions given on the package of orzo. Add corn a minute before draining the water.

3. Drain and rinse in cold water. Drain well and add into a bowl.

4. Add chicken, cilantro, and tomatoes and toss well. Scatter feta on top. Chill for a couple of hours.

5. Pour dressing on top. Toss well and serve.

24. Chicken Quinoa Bowl

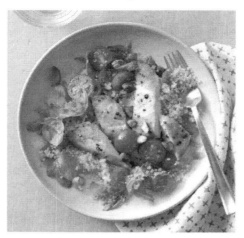

Nutritional values:

- Calories: 516
- Fat: 27 g
- Carbohydrate: 29 g
- Protein: 43 g

Ingredients:

- 1 boneless, skinless chicken breast half (about 3.5–4 ounces), cut into 1 inch cubes
- ¼ cup uncooked quinoa
- ½ small avocado, peeled, pitted, sliced
- 1 large egg, soft boiled, peeled, halved
- ½ tablespoon olive oil
- ½ cup water
- 1 cup arugula
- ¼ cup halved cherry tomatoes
- Pepper to taste
- ½ tablespoon sesame seeds
- Salt to taste

Directions:

1. Pour water into a saucepan and place it over high heat. When water starts boiling, add quinoa and stir.
2. Turn down the heat and cook covered until dry.
3. While the quinoa is cooking, place a pan over medium heat. Add oil. When oil is hot, add chicken and cook until brown all over.
4. Turn off the heat.
5. To serve: Place quinoa in a bowl. Scatter arugula over the quinoa followed by chicken and avocado.
6. Next scatter the tomatoes. Sprinkle sesame seeds on top. Place the egg halves on top and serve.

25. Sweet Potato and Broccoli Chicken

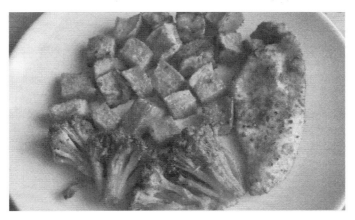

Nutritional values:

- Calories: 560
- Fat: 26 g
- Carbohydrate: 47 g
- Protein: 35 g

Ingredients:

- 1 boneless, chicken breast half (about 3.5–4 ounces)
- ½ cup cubed sweet potato
- 2 small cloves garlic, peeled, minced
- 1 ½ tablespoons chopped walnuts
- Salt to taste
- 1 cup broccoli florets
- Pepper to taste
- ¼ cup chopped red onion
- 1/8 cup dried cranberries
- 1 tablespoon olive oil

Directions:

1. Set the temperature of your oven to 375 °F and preheat the oven.
2. Prepare a baking sheet by lining it with parchment paper.
3. Place sweet potato, broccoli, garlic, and onion on the baking sheet. Sprinkle salt and pepper to taste. Trickle oil over the vegetables and mix well. Spread it evenly on one half of the baking sheet. Cover the baking sheet with foil and put the baking sheet in the oven.
4. Set the timer for 20 minutes. After baking for 8 minutes, place chicken on the other half of the baking sheet.
5. Continue baking for the remaining 12 minutes.
6. Now place cranberries and walnuts on the baking sheet. Continue baking until the chicken is well-cooked inside, about 8–9 minutes.
7. Serve.

26. Chicken Parmesan

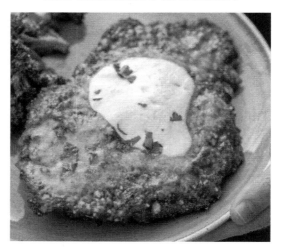

Nutritional values:

- Calories: 394

- Fat: 20.2 g

- Carbohydrate: 19.5 g

- Protein: 34.1 g

Ingredients:

- 1 skinless, boneless chicken breast half (4 ounces), trimmed

- 1/8 cup dried breadcrumbs (use whole-wheat breadcrumbs if possible)

- 2 teaspoons extra-virgin olive oil

- 1 small clove garlic, peeled, minced

- ¼ teaspoon Italian seasoning

- ¼ cup part-skim shredded mozzarella cheese

- Freshly ground pepper to taste

- ½ tablespoon freshly grated parmesan cheese

- ½ small onion, chopped

- ½ can (from a 14.1 ounces can) crushed tomatoes

- Salt to taste

- 1 tablespoon chopped fresh herbs of your choice

Directions:

1. Place chicken breast in between two sheets of cling wrap and beat with a meat mallet (from the smooth side) until it is about ¼ inch thick.

2. Season the chicken with pepper.

3. Mix together parmesan, breadcrumbs, and 1 teaspoon oil in a shallow bowl.

4. Set the oven to broil mode and preheat it to medium-high heat.

5. Pour remaining oil into an ovenproof skillet and place it over medium–high heat.

6. When oil is hot, place chicken in the pan and cook until the underside is golden brown. Turn the chicken over and cook the other side until golden brown. Remove chicken from the pan and place on a plate.

7. Drop garlic and onion into the same pan and cook for a couple of minutes until tender.

8. Add tomatoes, pepper, salt, and Italian seasoning and mix well. Stir often and cook for a couple of minutes.

9. Add chicken into the pan along with any cooked juices. Mix well. Turn the chicken around in the sauce so that it is well coated with the sauce.

10. Turn off the heat. Scatter mozzarella cheese over the chicken. Scatter breadcrumbs over the cheese. Place the pan in the oven and broil for a couple of minutes. Be careful to avoid burning.

11. Garnish with herbs and serve.

Fish and Seafood Recipes

Fish and seafood are rich in heart-healthy omega-3 fatty acids, lean protein, and a variety of other minerals and nutrients. Consuming seafood regularly is good for your overall health and wellbeing. So, get your dose of healthy omega-3 fatty acids and protein without increasing carb consumption with these delicious and healthy recipes.

27. Poached Fish in Tomato Basil Sauce

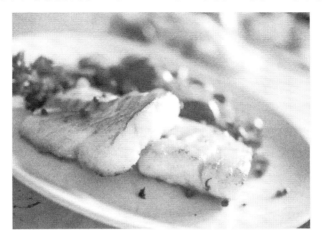

Nutritional values:

- Calories: 185
- Fat: 2 g
- Carbohydrate: 6 g
- Protein: 32 g

Ingredients:

- 1 frozen white fish filet (6 ounces)
- 1 small clove garlic, thinly sliced
- 1 tablespoon dry white wine
- Pepper to taste
- ½ cup halved cherry tomatoes
- 1/8 cup light chicken stock
- Salt to taste
- 1 tablespoon finely chopped basil leaves + extra to garnish

Directions:

1. Place a pan over medium heat. Add tomatoes, pepper, salt, and garlic and cook for a few minutes until tomatoes are slightly soft.

2. Pour white wine and stock and stir well. Add fish and basil and give it a good stir. Cover the pan and cook for about 18–20 minutes or until the fish is cooked through.

3. Garnish with some basil and serve with some cooked grains of your choice. The nutritional values of the grains are not included. You can even have it with a side of roast Brussels sprout or Sautéed Broccoli Stir Fry with Garlic (the recipe is included in the chapter for sides)

28. Lemon Roasted Salmon with Sweet Potatoes and Broccolini

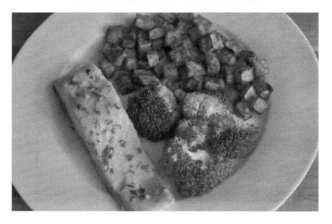

Nutritional values:

- Calories: 282
- Fat: 14.7 g
- Carbohydrate: 11.6 g
- Protein: 20.6 g

Ingredients:

- 3 ounces wild-caught salmon filets
- ½ medium sweet potato, cut into cubes
- 1/8 teaspoon ground cumin
- 1 cup broccolini or broccoli florets
- ½ tablespoon butter
- A pinch garlic powder
- Sea salt to taste
- Freshly ground black pepper to taste
- 1 tablespoon olive oil
- ½ tablespoon lemon juice
- Red pepper flakes to taste
- Chopped thyme to garnish

Directions:

1. Start off by preheating your oven to 425 °F.
2. Take a baking sheet and put the sweet potato cubes on one side of the baking sheet. Trickle ½ tablespoon oil. Sprinkle salt, cumin, and pepper over the sweet potatoes and toss well. Spread it in a single layer.
3. Place the baking sheet in the oven and set the timer for 15 minutes.
4. Meanwhile, add lemon juice, pepper flakes, salt, butter, pepper, and thyme in a microwave safe bowl. Heat in a microwave for about 15 seconds. Mix well.
5. Take another baking sheet and line it with foil. Grease the foil with cooking spray.
6. Put the salmon on the foil. Spoon the lemon sauce on the salmon.
7. Place broccolini on the other side of the baking sheet. Drizzle ½ tablespoon oil and mix well.
8. Sprinkle salt and pepper over the broccolini and toss well. Place the sweet potatoes along with the broccolini.
9. Put the baking sheet into the oven and set the timer for about 10 minutes. Check the salmon and broccolini after 10 minutes. If any one of these is cooked, take that out and continue baking until the other is cooked.
10. Serve hot. You can make this ahead of time and place them in meal prep containers in the refrigerator.

29. Fish Tacos

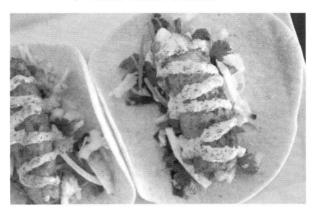

Nutritional values:

- Calories: 254
- Fat: 4 g
- Carbohydrate: 29 g
- Protein: 26 g

Ingredients:

- ½ tablespoon reduced-fat plain yogurt
- 1 tablespoon finely chopped cilantro, divided
- 1 small onion, chopped
- 4 ounces white fish like cod or mahi or halibut, rinsed, dried with paper towels
- 1 whole-wheat tortilla (6 inches)
- Lime wedge to serve (optional)
- 2 teaspoons fresh lime juice, divided
- ½ small tomato, chopped
- ¼ medium jalapeño, deseeded, chopped (optional)
- Salt to taste
- ¼ cup shredded cabbage

Directions:

1. You can grill the fish on a grill or in a broiler.
2. Set the grill or broiler to high heat and preheat it.
3. Combine yogurt, ½ tablespoon cilantro, and 1 teaspoon lime juice in a bowl.
4. To make salsa: Add onion, tomato, jalapeno, and remaining cilantro into a bowl and mix well. This is the salsa.
5. Sprinkle salt over the fish and place on the grill or in the broiler and cook for 4–5 minutes. Flip sides and cook the other side for 4–5 minutes or until the fish cooks well inside. It should flake readily when pierced with a fork.
6. Warm the tortilla following the directions given on the package.
7. To assemble: Place the tortilla on a plate. Place fish over the tortilla. Scatter cabbage over the fish. Trickle remaining lime juice and yogurt mixture.
8. Serve garnished with lime wedge along with salsa on the side.

30. Mediterranean Couscous with Tuna and Pepperoncini

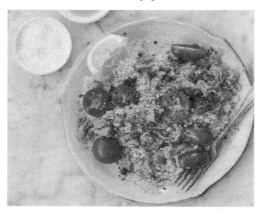

Nutritional values: Couscous + tuna and pepperoncini

- Calories: 226 + 193 = 419
- Fat: 1 g + 9 g = 10 g
- Carbohydrate: 44 g + 6 g = 52 g
- Protein: 8 g + 22 g = 30 g

Ingredients:

For couscous:

- ¼ cup chicken broth or water
- ¼ teaspoon salt or to taste
- 5 tablespoons couscous
- Extra-virgin olive oil to drizzle

For tuna:

- ½ can (from a 5 ounces can) oil packed tuna
- 1/8 cup sliced pepperoncini
- 1 tablespoon capers
- ½ cup halved cherry tomatoes
- 1 tablespoon chopped fresh parsley
- Lemon wedge to serve

Directions:

1. To make couscous: Pour broth into a small pot and place it over medium heat. When the broth starts boiling, turn off the heat. Add couscous and stir.

2. Keep the pot covered and let it rest for 10 minutes or until all the liquid is absorbed and the couscous is soft.

3. Fluff up the grains using a fork. Add salt and pepper to taste. Drizzle some oil as well.

4. Meanwhile, combine tomatoes, tuna, parsley, pepperoncini, and capers in a bowl and mix well.

5. Spread couscous on a serving plate. Place tuna mixture on top. Decorate with a lemon wedge and serve.

31. Teriyaki Shrimp Sushi Bowl

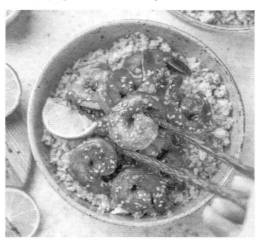

Nutritional values:
- Calories: 584
- Fat: 30 g
- Carbohydrate: 46 g
- Protein: 34 g

Ingredients:
- ½ cup cooked white rice
- ½ teaspoon olive oil
- 2 cloves garlic, peeled, minced
- ½ tablespoon sesame seeds
- ½ avocado, peeled, cut into slices
- ¼ cup cooked quinoa
- 4 ounces cooked shrimp, defrosted
- 1 tablespoon teriyaki sauce (recipe mentioned below)
- ¼ cup sliced cucumber

For teriyaki sauce:
- 1 tablespoon soy sauce
- ¾ tablespoon rice vinegar
- ¾ teaspoon cornstarch
- ½ tablespoon maple syrup
- 1/8 teaspoon grated fresh ginger

For spicy mayonnaise:

- ¼ teaspoon sriracha sauce or more to taste
- ½ tablespoon mayonnaise

Directions:
1. Pour oil into a small skillet and place it over medium heat. When oil is hot, add shrimp and heat it up well.
2. Meanwhile, mix up all the teriyaki sauce ingredients in a bowl.
3. Now stir the garlic into the skillet with shrimp and let it cook for a few seconds until you get a nice aroma.
4. Add a tablespoon of teriyaki sauce and mix well. Turn off the heat. Garnish with sesame seeds.
5. Place quinoa and rice in a serving bowl and mix well. Place shrimp on top. Scatter avocado and cucumber on top. Drizzle remaining teriyaki sauce on top and serve.
6. Combine mayonnaise and sriracha sauce in a bowl. Trickle the mayonnaise on top and serve.

32. Honey Soy Shrimp and Broccoli

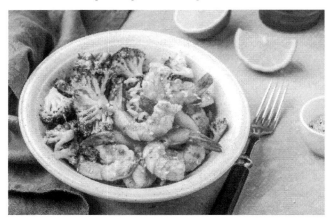

Nutritional values:

- Calories: 301
- Fat: 0.6 g
- Carbohydrate: 32 g
- Protein: 44 g

Ingredients:

- 1 ¼ tablespoons honey
- 1 teaspoon grated fresh ginger
- 1 clove garlic, diced
- 8 ounces extra-large shrimp, peeled, deveined, with tail on
- 1 tablespoon light soy sauce
- ¼ teaspoon red pepper flakes or to taste
- 1 ¼ cups broccoli florets
- Salt to taste

Directions:

1. Add honey, ginger, soy sauce, garlic, and red pepper flakes into a bowl and mix well.
2. Place shrimp in a bowl. Pour half the sauce mixture over the shrimp and toss well.
3. Cover the bowl with cling wrap and place it in the refrigerator for 20 minutes.
4. Meanwhile, pour enough water into a saucepan to cover at least 1 inch in height from the bottom of the saucepan.
5. Place a steamer basket in the saucepan.
6. Place the broccoli in the steamer basket and cover the saucepan with a lid.
7. Steam until the broccoli turns bright green. It should be crisp as well as tender.
8. Place a pan over medium heat. When the pan is hot, add shrimp into the pan and spread it all over the pan in a single layer. When the shrimp turns light pink in color, turn the shrimp over and cook for 2 to 3 minutes or until shrimp cooks.
9. Add broccoli into the pan. Pour remaining sauce mixture and mix well.
10. Serve hot. You can also cool it completely and transfer into a meal prep container. Make sure to keep it refrigerated.

33. Thai Coconut Curry Shrimp Noodle Bowls

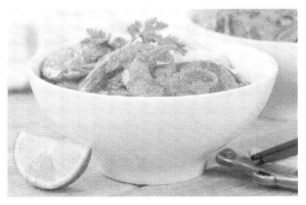

Nutritional values:

- Calories: 450
- Fat: 15 g
- Carbohydrate: 21 g
- Protein: 15 g

Ingredients:

- ¾ tablespoon coconut oil
- 1 small onion, sliced
- 1/8 orange bell pepper, sliced
- 1/8 red bell pepper, sliced
- 2 ounces raw, peeled, deveined shrimp
- Salt to taste
- 1 clove garlic, minced
- ½ tablespoon red curry paste
- 3.5 ounces canned light coconut milk
- 3.5 ounces canned, full-fat coconut milk
- Chopped cilantro to garnish
- Pepper to taste

- ¼ teaspoon freshly grated ginger
- 1/7 cup sugar snap peas
- 1.5 ounces cooked rice noodles or soba noodles
- 1/8 cup thinly sliced green onion

Directions:

1. Add ½ a tablespoon of oil into a pan and let it melt over medium heat.
2. When oil melts, drop the shrimp into the pan and spread it evenly in a single layer.
3. Add salt and pepper to taste. Transfer the shrimp into a bowl.
4. Pour remaining oil into the pan. Once oil is hot, add bell peppers, onion, pepper, and salt and mix well.
5. When the vegetables are slightly tender, stir in ginger, garlic, and curry paste.
6. Cook for a couple of minutes. Stir in snap peas and all of the coconut milk. Scrape the bottom of the pan to remove any browned bits.
7. When the mixture starts boiling, add the shrimp back into the pan. Add green onions and stir well. Heat thoroughly.
8. To assemble: Place noodles in a serving bowl. Pour shrimp curry on top. Garnish with cilantro and serve.

34. Salmon and Sweet Potato Grain Bowls

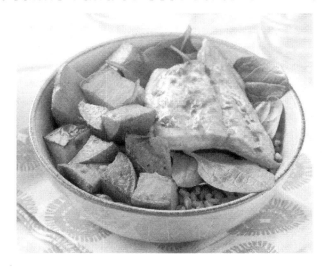

Nutritional values:

- Calories: 662
- Fat: 28.9 g
- Carbohydrate: 61.1 g
- Protein: 35.5 g

Ingredients:

- 1 tablespoon extra-virgin olive oil
- Salt to taste
- 1 salmon filet (4 ounces) skinless
- ½ cup warm cooked farro
- ½ tablespoon harissa or any other spice blend of your choice
- ½ pound sweet potato, peeled, cut into 1 inch cubes
- 1 cup baby spinach

Directions:

1. Set the temperature of your oven to 425 °F and preheat the oven. Prepare a baking sheet by spraying it with cooking spray.
2. Place harissa in a bowl. Add salt and oil and mix well. Stir in the sweet potato cubes.
3. Spread the sweet potatoes on the baking sheet and place it in the oven. Set the timer for 20 minutes or bake until nearly tender.
4. Now place the salmon in the same bowl and turn it around in the bowl to coat any leftover mixture.
5. Now place salmon on the baking sheet along with sweet potato and bake for 6–8 minutes or until the fish cooks and the sweet potato cubes are tender.
6. If you do not want to use farro, you can use any other cooked grains of your choice like quinoa or rice etc. add spinach and farro into a bowl and mix well. Cover the bowl and let the spinach wilt.
7. Place sweet potato in the bowl, over the farro. Place salmon on top and serve.

35. Spring Salad with Tarragon Vinaigrette

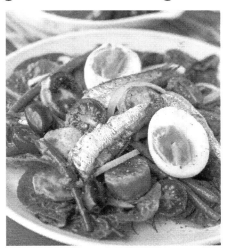

Nutritional values:

- Calories: 358
- Fat: 26.1 g
- Carbohydrate: 8.8 g
- Protein: 22.8 g

Ingredients:

For the dressing:

- 1 tablespoon red wine vinegar or any other vinegar
- ½ teaspoon whole-grain mustard
- Salt to taste
- ½ clove garlic, grated or minced
- 1 tablespoon extra-virgin olive oil
- 1/8 teaspoon dried tarragon
- Freshly ground pepper to taste

For the salad:

- ¼ bunch asparagus, trim the hard ends
- ½ bag (from a 5 ounces bag) mixed salad greens
- ½ can (from a 4 ounces can) sardines
- 1 large hard boiled egg, peeled, quartered
- 5 cherry tomatoes
- 3 olives, pitted, sliced (optional)

Directions:

1. To make dressing: Add vinegar, mustard, salt, garlic, oil, tarragon, and pepper in a bowl and whisk well. Cover and keep it aside for a few minutes for the flavors to meld.

2. Blanch the asparagus in a pot of boiling water for about 3 minutes. Drain and rinse in cold water. Drain once again.

3. Place mixed greens on a plate. Scatter asparagus, sardines, tomatoes, olives and egg over the greens. Drizzle the dressing over the salad and serve.

36. Salsa Spaghetti with Sardines

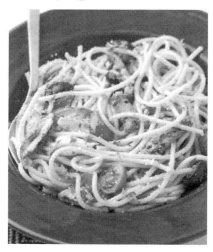

Nutritional values:

- Calories: 442
- Fat: 16 g
- Carbohydrate: 43 g
- Protein: 31 g

Ingredients:

- 1.75 ounces whole-wheat spaghetti
- ½ onion, minced
- ¼ teaspoon finely chopped red chili
- 2 tablespoons thinly sliced fresh basil or ½ teaspoon chopped fresh oregano
- 1 large tomato, very finely chopped
- 2 black olives, pitted, quartered
- 1 tablespoon lemon juice
- ¼ teaspoon grated lemon zest
- 1 can (4 ounces) sardines in olive oil, drained but retain the oil
- Salt to taste
- Pepper juice

Directions:

1. Follow the directions given on the package of spaghetti and cook the spaghetti.
2. Place tomatoes, olives, lemon zest, chili, and basil in a bowl.
3. Warm the sardines in a microwave or a pan.
4. Chop sardines into chunks. Add sardines and tomato mixture to spaghetti. Add pepper, lemon juice and a little drained oil from the can of sardines and toss well.
5. Transfer onto a plate and serve.

37. Chickpea Tuna Lettuce Wraps

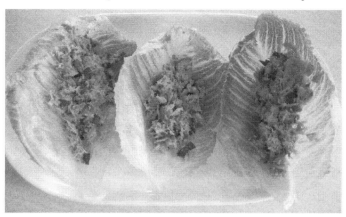

Nutritional values:

- Calories: 324
- Fat: 9 g
- Carbohydrate: 33 g
- Protein: 30 g

Ingredients:

- ½ cup cooked chickpeas
- 3 large lettuce leaves, preferably butter lettuce
- ½ small onion, chopped
- 1 tablespoon chopped cilantro
- Juice of ½ lemon
- ½ tablespoon tahini or mayonnaise
- ½ can (from a 6 ounces can) tuna in water, drained
- ½ medium carrot, chopped
- ½ stalk celery, chopped
- ½ clove garlic, peeled, minced
- Pepper to taste
- 1 tablespoon Dijon mustard
- Salt to taste

Directions:

1. Place chickpeas in the food processor bowl. Give short pulses until it is chunky.

2. Transfer chickpeas into a bowl. Add tuna, onion, cilantro, carrot, celery, and garlic and mix well.

3. Divide the mixture among the lettuce leaves. Wrap and serve. You can use tortilla or pita bread instead of lettuce leaves to increase the calorie intake.

38. Salmon with Creamy Smashed Potatoes

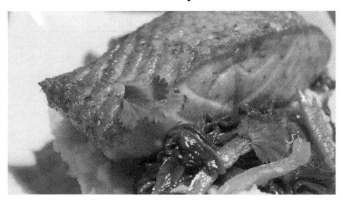

Nutritional values:

- Calories: 409
- Fat: 18 g
- Carbohydrate: 23 g
- Protein: 36 g

Ingredients:

- 4 ounces baby potatoes
- ¾ teaspoon olive oil
- ¾ tablespoon heavy cream
- Salt to taste
- White pepper to taste
- Flaky sea salt to garnish
- ½ green onion or spring onion or scallion, thinly sliced
- ¾ tablespoon prepared horseradish
- 1 salmon filet with skin (5 ounces)
- 2 teaspoons lemon juice or to taste

Directions:

1. Boil potatoes in a small pot of water until fork tender. Drain and smash the potatoes with the back of a fork. Place them in a bowl.

2. Combine horseradish and cream in a bowl. Add half this mixture to the potatoes. Add salt, pepper, and spring onions and mix well. Cover and keep it aside.

3. Dry the salmon filet with paper towels.

4. Sprinkle salt over the salmon.

5. Pour oil into a heavy skillet and let it heat over high heat. When oil is hot, place the salmon in the pan, with the skin side facing down.

6. Cook for 3 minutes. Turn the salmon over and cook the other side for 1 minute.

7. Turn off the heat. Place potatoes on a serving plate. Spoon the remaining horseradish cream over the potatoes.

8. Place salmon over the potatoes, with the skin side facing on top. Sprinkle lemon zest over the salmon. Top with flaky sea salt and serve.

39. Shrimp and Avocado Quinoa Bowl

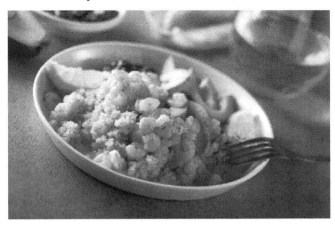

Nutritional values:

- Calories: 458
- Fat: 22 g
- Carbohydrate: 63 g
- Protein: 33 g

Ingredients:

- 4 ounces raw shrimp, peeled, deveined
- ¼ medium cucumber, peeled, diced
- ½ teaspoon olive oil
- 1 clove garlic, peeled, minced
- ½ tablespoon lime juice
- Pepper to taste
- ½ tablespoon butter
- ½ tablespoon honey
- Salt to taste
- ½ cup cooked quinoa
- ½ small avocado, peeled, pitted, sliced

Directions:

1. Add oil and butter into a skillet and let it heat over medium heat.
2. Once butter melts, drop the shrimp into the pan and spread it in a single layer.
3. When the underside is cooked, turn sides and cook the other side as well.
4. Season with salt and pepper. Add honey and lime juice and stir. Turn off the heat.
5. Serve quinoa in bowls topped with shrimp, cucumber, and avocado.

40. Shrimp Pad Thai

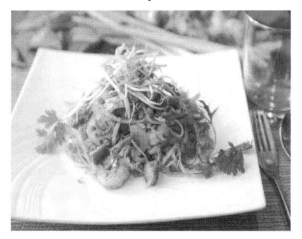

Nutritional values:

- Calories: 462
- Fat: 16.1 g
- Carbohydrate: 64.3 g
- Protein: 15.8 g

Ingredients:

For sauce mixture:

- ½ tablespoon brown sugar
- ½ tablespoon fish sauce
- 1 teaspoon Sriracha sauce
- ¼ cup chopped green onions (chopped into 2 inch pieces)
- 1 clove garlic, peeled, minced
- 2 ounces Thai flat rice noodles or any other flat noodles
- ½ tablespoon low- sodium soy sauce
- 1 teaspoon fresh lime juice
- ¾ tablespoon canola oil
- 2 ounces peeled, deveined large shrimp

To serve:

- 1 tablespoon roasted peanuts, unsalted
- ¼ cup bean sprouts
- 2 teaspoons fresh basil, chopped

Directions:

1. Follow the directions given on the package of noodles and cook the noodles.
2. Mix together brown sugar, soy sauce, fish sauce, lime juice, and Sriracha sauce in a bowl.
3. Place a wok or skillet over medium-high heat. Add oil. When oil is hot, add onion, garlic, and shrimp and sauté for a couple of minutes or until the shrimp is nearly cooked.
4. Add noodles, mix well. Add the sauce mixture. Mix well.
5. Place noodles in a bowl. Scatter bean sprouts, peanuts, and basil over the noodles and serve.

Beef and Pork Recipes

Beef and pork are excellent sources of healthy protein and fats needed for your body's overall functioning. Also, these animal proteins are incredibly versatile and can be cooked in different ways. Add a portion of salad or a side of your choice to these recipes and a hearty meal will be ready within no time!

41. Skillet Pepper Steak

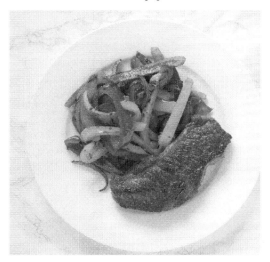

Nutritional values:

- Calories: 226
- Fat: 11 g
- Carbohydrate: 12 g
- Protein: 21 g

Ingredients:

- 3 ounces top round beef, cut into thin slices
- 1 ½ teaspoons peanut oil or any other oil of your choice
- ¾ teaspoon rice wine vinegar
- ¼ red bell pepper, cut into thin slices
- ¼ green bell pepper, cut into thin slices
- ¼ yellow bell pepper, cut into thin slices
- ¼ orange bell pepper, cut into thin slices
- 1 clove garlic, minced
- Sesame seeds to garnish
- Kosher salt to taste
- ¾ teaspoon soy sauce
- ¼ teaspoon crushed red pepper flakes
- ¼ bunch scallions, thinly sliced
- Freshly ground black pepper to taste

Directions:

1. Sprinkle salt and pepper over the steak.

2. Pour half the oil into a skillet and place the skillet over medium-high heat.

3. When oil is hot, add the steak into the bowl and cook until the underside is brown. Turn the steak over and cook the other side for 2 minutes but not well-cooked inside.

4. Remove steak from the pan and keep it in a bowl.

5. Drizzle vinegar and soy sauce over the steak. Add red pepper flakes and mix well.

6. Pour remaining oil into the skillet. When oil is hot add all the bell pepper slices into the pan and sauté for a few minutes until slightly tender. Make sure the bell peppers have a crunch in them.

7. Move the bell peppers on one part of the pan. Add the steak into the middle of the skillet. Let it cook for a couple of minutes.

8. Add garlic and mix well. Mix up the steak with the bell peppers.

9. Scatter sesame seeds and scallions on top and serve right away. Serve steak with bread or potatoes or macaroni and cheese or any other favorite grains of your choice. The nutritional value of which is not included in the recipe. You can also serve with Sautéed broccoli stir fry with garlic or roasted Brussels sprouts, the recipes are given in the chapter Side and Snack recipes.

42. Sheet Pan Marinated Steak Tips with Veggies

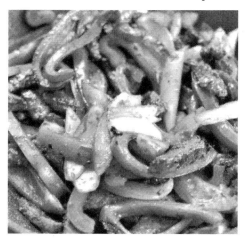

Nutritional values:

- Calories: 368

- Fat: 21.8 g

- Carbohydrate: 21 g

- Protein: 26.8 g

Ingredients:

For marinade:

- 1 ½ tablespoons balsamic vinegar

- ¼ teaspoon chopped rosemary

- Black pepper to taste

- 1 ½ tablespoons olive oil

- ¼ teaspoon Dijon mustard

- 1 small clove garlic, minced

- Salt to taste

For steak and vegetables:

- 4 ounces sirloin steak tips (about 1 ½ inches diameter)

- ½ cup halved or quartered baby potatoes

- ½ teaspoon avocado oil, divided

- ¼ red bell pepper, deseeded, cut into slices

- ¼ zucchini or summer squash, cut into ¼ inch thick round slices

- 1 small red onion, cut into ¼ inch thick round slices

- Salt to taste

- Pepper to taste

- ¼ bunch asparagus, cut into 2 inch pieces

Directions:

1. To make marinade: Combine vinegar, rosemary, pepper, garlic, salt, and Dijon mustard in a bowl. Whisk well.

2. Whisking constantly, pour oil in a thin drizzle. Keep whisking until the marinade is emulsified.

3. To prepare steak and vegetables: Place steak tips in a bowl. Drizzle about half the marinade over the steak tips. Mix well and keep it aside for a while.

4. Start off by preheating your oven to 400 °F.

5. Prepare a baking sheet by greasing it with some cooking spray.

6. Place potatoes along with onions in a bowl. Drizzle half the oil over it and sprinkle salt to taste.

7. Spread the mixture on the baking sheet. Place the baking sheet in the oven and set the timer for 10 minutes.

8. Combine asparagus, zucchini, bell peppers, and salt in a bowl. Drizzle remaining oil over the vegetables. Toss well.

9. Spread it on the baking sheet along with the onions and potatoes and let it bake for about 10 minutes. Take out the baking sheet.

10. Turn on the broiler and let it preheat to high heat for about 5 minutes.

11. Take out only the steak from the marinade and place it on the baking sheet. Make some space on the baking sheet by keeping the vegetables together.

12. The remaining marinade is no more needed. Place the baking sheet in the oven and let it broil for a few minutes, about 5 minutes. Turn the steak tips over and let it broil for about 3 minutes or until cooked as per your preference.

13. Once it is cooked take out the baking sheet and let it sit for about 10 minutes.

14. Place on a plate. Pour remaining marinade on top and serve.

43. Cheeseburger Skillet

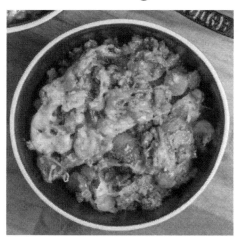

Nutritional values:

- Calories: 325

- Fat: 16 g

- Carbohydrate: 6 g

- Protein: 30 g

Ingredients:

- 1 slice center cut bacon, cut into strips

- 4 ounces ground beef

- ½ tablespoon light mayonnaise

- ½ tablespoon pickle juice

- 2 ounces shredded cheese

- 1 tablespoon sugar-free ketchup

- ½ tablespoon Dijon mustard or whole-grain mustard

- ¾ teaspoon Worcestershire sauce

- Salt to taste

- Pepper to taste

- 3 ounces radishes, trimmed, quartered

- Dill pickle chips to garnish

- Chopped parsley to garnish (optional)

Directions:

1. Place bacon in a pan and place it over medium-high heat. Cook until crisp. Remove bacon with a slotted spoon and place on a plate. When bacon cools down, crumble into smaller pieces.

2. Add radishes into the pan and sauté until they are slightly soft.

3. Move the radishes to one edge of the pan and place the beef in the center. Cook until brown. As you stir the meat, break into smaller pieces. When the meat gets cooked, turn off the heat.

4. Meanwhile, combine mayonnaise, ketchup, pickle juice, mustard, and Worcestershire sauce in a bowl.

5. Preheat your oven to 400 °F.

6. Add meat mixture into the sauce and mix well. Transfer the mixture into a small baking dish.

7. Spread cheese on top. Place dill pickle chips on top.

8. Place the baking dish in the oven and set the timer for about 5 minutes or until the cheese melts.

9. Garnish with bacon and parsley. Sprinkle salt and pepper on top and serve it with mashed sweet potatoes or roasted vegetables (the recipe is given in the chapter Side and Snack Recipes)

44. Egg Roll Bowls

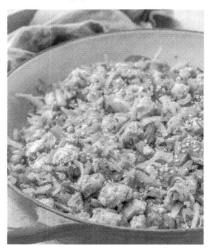

Nutritional values:

- Calories: 233
- Fat: 7.1 g
- Carbohydrate: 12.9 g
- Protein: 28.9 g

Ingredients:

- ¼ teaspoon olive oil
- ½ small onion, diced
- 1 small clove garlic, minced
- 3.5 ounces coleslaw mix
- ¾ teaspoon rice vinegar
- 4 ounces ground beef or pork
- ¼ inch fresh ginger, peeled, minced
- ½ carrot, peeled, shredded
- ¾ tablespoon tamari or coconut aminos or soy sauce
- ¼–½ teaspoon toasted sesame oil
- ¾ teaspoon rice vinegar or cider vinegar
- 1/8 cup sliced green onion

Directions:

1. Pour oil into a skillet and let it heat over medium heat. When oil is hot, add meat and cook until brown. You can use ground chicken or turkey instead of pork or beef. As you stir, break the meat into smaller pieces.

2. Stir in the onion and cook until slightly soft. Stir in ginger and garlic. Keep stirring for a few seconds or up to a minute, until you get a nice aroma.

3. Mix in the carrots and the coleslaw mixture. Add vinegar and tamari and mix well. Once cabbage turns limp, add green onion and sesame oil. Mix well and turn off the heat.

4. Transfer into a bowl and serve hot.

45. Pork Chops and Vegetables

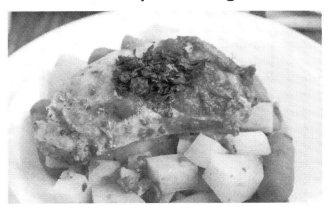

Nutritional values:

- Calories: 345
- Fat: 7 g
- Carbohydrate: 32 g
- Protein: 36 g

Ingredients:

- ¾ teaspoon butter
- 1 ½ tablespoons beef broth
- 1 carrot, cut into 1 inch pieces
- 1 clove garlic, minced
- Salt and pepper to taste
- 1 pork loin chop (about 6 ounces and 1 inch thick)
- 1 medium potato, cut into bite size cubes
- 1 large onion, diced into bite size pieces
- 1 tablespoon chopped parsley

Directions:

1. Place a pan over medium-high heat. Spray the pan with cooking spray. Add butter and allow it to melt.

2. Season the pork chop with salt and pepper and place in the pan. Cook for about 3 minutes on each side.

3. Stir in broth, carrot, potato, garlic, and onion. Add salt and pepper to taste.

4. When the mixture starts boiling, turn down the heat to low heat. Cover the pan and cook until the vegetables and pork are cooked through.

5. Garnish with parsley and serve.

46. Lentil Kielbasa Soup

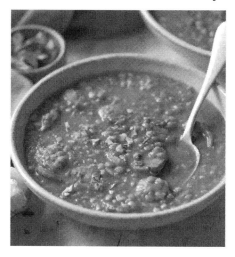

Nutritional values:

- Calories: 689
- Fat: 35 g
- Carbohydrate: 61 g
- Protein: 34 g

Ingredients:

- ½ tablespoon extra-virgin olive oil
- ½ celery stalk sliced
- ¼ small onion, chopped
- ¼ cup French lentils or green lentils
- 4 ½ cups chicken broth
- ½ head broccoli rabe, chopped
- 3 ounces kielbasa, sliced
- 1 small carrot, peeled, chopped
- 1 clove garlic, sliced
- ¼ can (from a 15 ounces can) crushed tomatoes
- Kosher salt to taste
- Freshly ground pepper to taste

Directions:

1. Pour oil into a pot and let it heat over medium heat. Once the oil is hot, add kielbasa and cook undisturbed until the underside is brown. Turn it over and cook the other side until brown.

2. Remove it onto a plate. Next add onion, carrot, celery, and garlic and cook until the vegetables are slightly tender.

3. Stir in lentils, broth, tomatoes, salt, pepper and kielbasa. Turn down the heat to low heat and cook covered until the lentils are cooked.

4. Add broccoli rabe and turn off the heat.

5. Serve hot. You can make this ahead of time and store it in the refrigerator after it is cooled, in an airtight container. Make sure to use it within 3 to 4 days.

47. Pistachio Crusted Pork Tenderloin with Apple and Escarole Salad

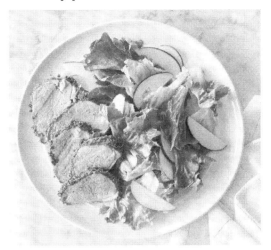

Nutritional values: Pork + Salad

- Calories: 381 +153 = 534
- Fat: 20 g + 14 g = 34 g
- Carbohydrate: 9 g + 8 g = 17 g
- Protein: 41 g + 1 g = 42 g

Ingredients:

For the pork:

- ¼ cup unsalted, shelled pistachios
- ½ teaspoon chopped fresh rosemary leaves
- 6 ounces pork tenderloin
- ½ clove garlic, peeled, minced
- Cayenne pepper to taste
- Kosher salt to taste
- Freshly ground black pepper to taste

For the salad:

- ¼ head escarole, torn into bite size pieces
- 1 teaspoon fresh lemon juice or more to taste
- ½ teaspoon Dijon mustard
- Kosher salt to taste
- Freshly ground black pepper to taste
- ¼ apple, cored, cut into thin slices
- ½ tablespoon white wine vinegar
- 1 tablespoon extra-virgin olive oil

Directions:

1. To make pork: The first thing to do is to preheat your oven to 375 °F.

2. Prepare a baking sheet by greasing it with some cooking spray.

3. Place pistachios, rosemary, garlic, and cayenne pepper in the small blender. Give short pulses until finely ground.

4. Transfer onto a plate.

5. Sprinkle salt and pepper over the pork chop. Roll the pork chop over the pistachio mixture.

6. Place the pork chop on the baking sheet and place it in the oven. Set the timer for about 25 minutes or cook as per your preference. The outer crust should be golden brown, preferably.

7. Take out the baking sheet from the oven and cover it loosely with foil.

8. Meanwhile make the salad: Combine apple, escarole, apple, and lemon juice in a bowl.

9. Add vinegar, mustard, salt, and pepper and toss well.

10. When the pork cools slightly, cut into slices of about ½ inch thick.

11. Place pork over the salad and serve.

48. Steak and Potatoes

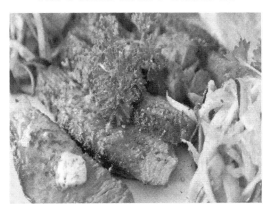

Nutritional values:

- Calories: 415
- Fat: 20.8 g
- Carbohydrate: 21.5 g
- Protein: 35.1 g

Ingredients:

- 4 ounces potatoes, cut into wedges of ½ inch thick
- Salt to taste
- 1 cup chopped asparagus
- 1/8 teaspoon garlic powder
- ¾ tablespoon crumbled blue cheese
- 1 ½ teaspoons extra-virgin olive oil, divided
- Pepper to taste
- 5 ounces skirt steak, trimmed
- 1/8 teaspoon dried rosemary

Directions:

1. Set the temperature of your oven to 425 °F and preheat the oven.
2. Prepare a baking sheet by spraying it with cooking spray.
3. Place potatoes in a bowl. Drizzle half the oil over the potatoes. Sprinkle salt and pepper and toss well.
4. Transfer the potatoes onto the prepared baking sheet and spread it evenly.
5. Place the baking sheet in the oven and set the timer for 15 minutes.
6. Place asparagus in the bowl. Drizzle remaining oil over the asparagus and toss well. Sprinkle salt and pepper over the asparagus and spread it on the baking sheet along with the potatoes.
7. Season the steak with rosemary, salt, garlic powder, and pepper and place over the vegetables.
8. Place the baking sheet in the oven and continue roasting until the steak is cooked through and the potatoes and asparagus are cooked. It should take another 10–15 minutes.
9. Place steak on a plate. Add blue cheese to the vegetables and stir. Place vegetables on the plate with steak and serve.

49. Flank Steak Gyros with Quick Pickles

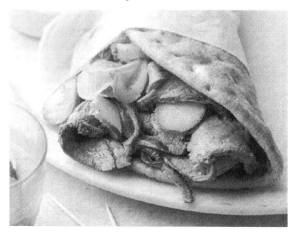

Nutritional values:

- Calories: 465
- Fat: 18 g
- Carbohydrate: 45 g
- Protein: 33 g

Ingredients:

For quick pickles:

- 1/8 cup white vinegar
- ¾ cup mixed vegetables like turnip, radish, and cucumber
- ¼ cup water
- ¼ teaspoon white sugar

For the steak:

- 1 ½ teaspoons extra-virgin olive oil, divided
- ¼ teaspoon ground cumin
- ¼ teaspoon ground coriander
- Salt to taste
- 4 ounces flank steak, trimmed
- ¼ teaspoons dried thyme
- Pepper to taste
- ¼ large onion, sliced

To serve:

- 2 tablespoons mayonnaise or tzatziki sauce or hummus
- 1 whole-wheat pita (6 inches), warmed

Directions:

1. Place the rack in the upper third position in the oven. Set the oven to broiler mode and let it preheat to high heat.

2. Prepare a baking sheet by lining it with aluminum foil.

3. Add half the oil, cumin, coriander, thyme, pepper, and salt into a bowl. Stir until well combined.

4. Rub this mixture on the steak, on both the sides. Place steak on the baking sheet.

5. Add onions into a bowl. Pour remaining oil and pepper over the onions. Place the onions all around the steak on the baking sheet.

6. Place the baking sheet in the oven. Broil for 10–15 minutes or until it is cooked. Stir once halfway through broiling. When meat is cooked, a meat thermometer when inserted in the thickest part of the meat should show 145 °F and the onions should be lightly charred.

7. Meanwhile, make the pickles: Add water, vinegar, sugar, and salt into a saucepan. Place the saucepan over medium heat.

8. When the mixture starts boiling, stir in the vegetables and let it cook for a minute. Turn off the heat.

9. Remove the steak from the oven and place on your cutting board. When cool enough to handle, slice the steak.

10. Drain the liquid in the saucepan. Make a slit on one end of the pita to make a pocket.

11. Place steak, pickled vegetables and onions in the pita pocket and serve with tzatziki sauce or mayonnaise or hummus.

50. Beef fajitas

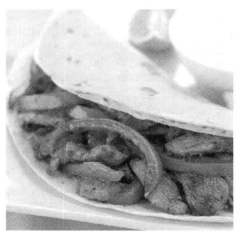

Nutritional values:

- Calories: 412
- Fat: 19 g
- Carbohydrate: 24 g
- Protein: 35 g

Ingredients:

- 4 ounces steak, cut into ½ inch thick strips
- ½ large bell pepper, cut into slices
- ½ small onion, sliced
- Juice of ½ lemon
- ½ tablespoon olive oil
- 1 ½ tablespoons low-sodium soy sauce
- ½ teaspoon chili powder
- 2 small corn tortillas

Directions:

1. Combine soy sauce, chili powder, lemon juice, and oil in a bowl. Place steak strips in a bowl.

2. Pour half the sauce mixture over the steak. Turn the beef strips around in the sauce mixture to coat well.

3. Add onion and bell pepper to the remaining sauce mixture. Set aside the steak and vegetables for about 20 minutes.

4. Place a skillet over medium heat. Add steak and cook until brown. Take out the steak from the pan and place on a plate.

5. Add onion and bell pepper along with sauce mixture into the pan. Cook for about 4–5 minutes or until tender.

6. Distribute the meat, onion, and bell pepper among the tortillas.

7. Serve.

51. Jalapeño Popper Burgers

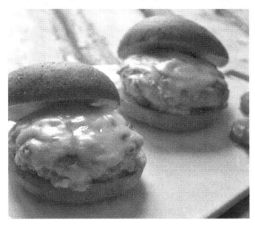

Nutritional values:

- Calories: 458
- Fat: 23.5 g
- Carbohydrate: 28.6 g
- Protein: 32.8 g

Ingredients:

- 0.75 ounce reduced-fat cream cheese, softened
- ¼ medium jalapeño pepper, deseeded, chopped
- Salt to taste
- 1 tablespoon ketchup
- 3 tablespoons shredded spicy cheese like pepper Jack cheese etc.
- 4 ounces ground sirloin
- 1 whole-wheat hamburger bun
- Toppings of your choice (optional)

Directions:

1. Add cream cheese, jalapeño, and cheese into a bowl and mix well. As you mix, mash them up together.
2. Make a ball of the mixture and flatten it into a circle of about 3 inches diameter.
3. You can cook the burger on a grill or in a pan.
4. Shape the meat into a burger of about 4 inches diameter and ½ inch in thickness. Sprinkle salt over the burger.
5. Cook the burger on the grill or in the pan for about 4 minutes on each side. The internal temperature of the cooked burger should show 160 °F on a meat thermometer.
6. Now place the cream cheese disc over the burger and cook for a couple of minutes until the cheese disc starts melting.
7. To serve: Toast the burger to the desired doneness on one side or both sides, as per your preference.
8. Drizzle ketchup over the burger. Place the burger on the bottom half of the bun. Cover with the top half of the bun and serve. You can serve with any toppings of your choice if desired. The nutritional values of the toppings are not included in the recipe.

52. Pork and Bok Choy Stir—Fry

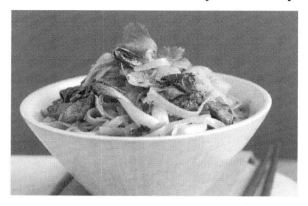

Nutritional values:

- Calories: 373
- Fat: 6 g
- Carbohydrate: 50.9 g
- Protein: 28.6 g

Ingredients:

- 2 ounces soba noodles or rice noodles
- 1 ½ tablespoons water
- ½ tablespoon soy sauce
- ¾ teaspoon canola oil or any cooking oil
- 4 ounces Bok Choy, trimmed, cut into thin long strips
- Chili garlic sauce to taste
- 4 ounces pork tenderloin, trimmed, cut into thin round slices
- 1 tablespoon rice wine or dry sherry
- ½ teaspoon cornstarch
- 1 small onion, thinly sliced
- 1 clove garlic, peeled, minced

Directions:

1. Cook the noodles following the directions given on the package.
2. Cut the round pork slices into thin strips, like matchsticks.
3. Combine water, soy sauce, rice wine, and cornstarch in a bowl. Keep it aside.
4. Pour oil into a skillet and let it heat over medium heat. When oil is hot, add onion and cook until onion turns translucent.
5. Stir in Bok Choy and cook for 3 to 4 minutes, until slightly tender.
6. Stir in garlic, pork, and chili garlic sauce. In 2–3 minutes the pork should be cooked. Stir often until pork is cooked.
7. Stir the cornstarch mixture once again and pour it into the pan. Keep stirring until the sauce is thick. Turn off the heat.
8. To serve: Place noodles in a serving bowl. Spoon the pork and vegetables along with sauce over the noodles and serve.
9. You can serve the pork and vegetables over rice or any other grains of your choice. The nutritional values will change if you use any other grains.

53. Pork Steaks with Roasted Summer Squash Salsa

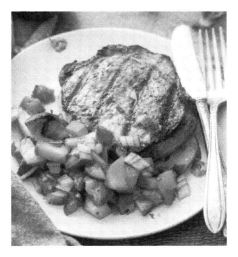

Nutritional values:

- Calories: 204
- Fat: 6 g
- Carbohydrate: 10 g
- Protein: 26 g

Ingredients:

For roasted summer squash salsa:

- 2 small tomatoes, cored, halved horizontally, deseeded
- 1 small red onion, halved horizontally
- ¼ zucchini, cut lengthwise into ¼ inch slices
- ¼ summer squash, cut lengthwise into ¼ inch slices
- ½ small jalapeño pepper, deseeded, halved lengthwise
- ¾ teaspoon olive oil
- 1/8 cup finely chopped fresh cilantro
- 1 small clove garlic, crushed
- 1 tablespoon fresh lime juice

For the pork:

- 1 pork tenderloin steak (4 ounces)
- Pepper to taste
- Salt to taste
- Olive oil cooking spray

Directions:

1. To make salsa: Set the temperature of your oven to 425 °F and preheat the oven.

2. Grease a roasting pan with cooking spray. Place the tomatoes with their cut side down in the pan. Also place onion, zucchini, jalapeño and squash in the pan in a single layer, without overlapping.

3. Set the timer for 10–12 minutes. Flip sides of the vegetables half way through roasting. When done, remove the roasting pan from the oven and set aside to cool.

4. Add lime juice, garlic, oil, cilantro, salt, and pepper into a bowl. Whisk well and set aside for a while for the flavors to infuse.

5. Peel the skin of the roasted tomato and place it on your cutting board.

6. Chop the tomatoes into smaller pieces and add into a bowl. Chop the vegetables into smaller pieces and add them into the bowl of tomatoes.

7. Pour the lime juice mixture into the bowl of vegetables and mix well. Cover the bowl and set aside until the pork is cooked.

8. Place a nonstick pan over medium high heat. Spray with cooking spray. Let it heat.

9. Season pork with salt and pepper and place in the pan. Cook for 3—4 minutes. Turn the pork over and cook the other side for 3—4 minutes. Turn off the heat.

10. Serve steak on a plate. Serve with salsa.

54. Orecchiette Pasta

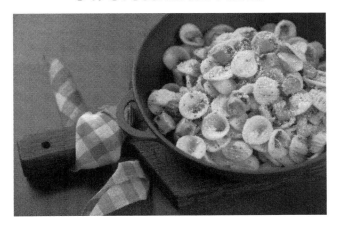

Nutritional values:

- Calories: 662

- Fat: 39.1 g

- Carbohydrate: 46.2 g

- Protein: 31.2 g

Ingredients:

- 1 tablespoon olive oil

- Salt to taste

- 1 ¾ cups low-sodium chicken broth, divided or more if required

- ¼ cup chopped arugula

- ¼ cup diced onion

- 4 ounces spicy Italian sausages, discard casings

- ½ cup + 1/8 cup orecchiette pasta

- 1/8 cup finely grated parmesan cheese

Directions:

1. Pour oil into a skillet and let it heat over medium heat. When oil is hot, add onion and a bit of salt and cook until onions are caramelized. Stir occasionally.

2. Add sausage and cook until brown. As you stir the sausage, break it into smaller pieces.

3. Add broth and stir. Scrape the bottom of the pan to remove any browned bits.

4. Stir in orecchiette pasta. Cook until pasta is al dente and nearly dry. In case the pasta is not cooked, and there is no liquid in the pan, add some more broth or water.

5. Add arugula and stir. Turn off the heat. Let it sit for a few minutes until arugula wilts.

6. Serve in a bowl topped with parmesan cheese.

Vegetarian Recipes and Salads

Vegetables are an excellent source of dietary fiber, minerals, and nutrients. These wholesome ingredients must be a part of your daily diet to ensure your body gets its essential dose of micros. From salads to wraps and stews, you will be introduced to a variety of healthy and mouth-watering vegetarian recipes!

55. Greek Couscous Salad

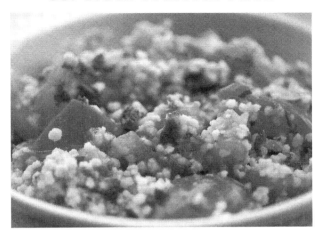

Nutritional values:

- Calories: 378
- Fat: 25.9 g
- Carbohydrate: 31.2 g
- Protein: 9 g

Ingredients:

For the salad:

- ½ package (from a 4.7 ounces) package pearled couscous mix with roasted garlic and olive oil
- ¼ green bell pepper, coarsely chopped
- ¼ red bell pepper, coarsely chopped
- ¼ yellow bell pepper, coarsely chopped
- ¼ cup halved cherry tomatoes
- ½ can (from a 15 ounces) chickpeas, drained, rinsed
- 1 teaspoon fresh lemon juice
- ¼ English cucumber, coarsely chopped
- 1 small red onion, chopped
- ¼ cup finely chopped flat-leaf parsley
- 1 tablespoon feta cheese

For the dressing:

- 1 tablespoon red wine vinegar
- 1 teaspoon fresh lemon juice or to taste
- ¼ teaspoon dried oregano
- Sea salt to taste
- 2 tablespoons olive oil
- Freshly cracked pepper to taste
- 1 small clove garlic, minced
- 1/8 teaspoon Dijon mustard

Directions:

1. Follow the directions given on the package of couscous and prepare the couscous. You are to add the seasoning mix that comes along with it.

2. Place onion in a bowl. Add lemon juice and stir. Let it rest for about 10 minutes.

3. To make dressing: Add all the dressing ingredients into a small jar. Fasten the lid and shake it vigorously until well combined. Let it sit for a while for the flavors to meld.

4. Combine couscous, chickpeas, vegetables, and feta cheese in a bowl and toss well. Add more lemon juice if required.

5. Pour dressing on top. Mix well and serve.

56. Vegan Quinoa Salad

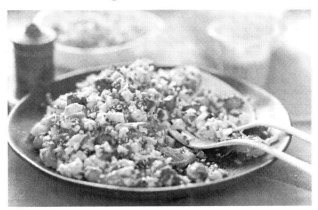

Nutritional values:

- Calories: 304
- Fat: 8.5 g
- Carbohydrate: 51.2 g
- Protein: 12.4 g

Ingredients:

For salad:

- ¼ cup dry quinoa
- ¼ cup edamame
- ¼ English cucumber, chopped
- ¼ cup chopped carrots
- 1/8 cup diced red onion
- ¼ can (from a 15 ounces can) chickpeas, drained, rinsed
- ¼ yellow bell pepper, chopped
- 4–5 cherry tomatoes, halved
- 1/8 cup chopped parsley (optional)

For the dressing:

- 1 clove garlic, minced
- ½ tablespoon Dijon mustard or stone ground mustard
- Salt to taste
- Juice of ½ lemon
- ½ tablespoon extra-virgin olive oil
- Pepper to taste

Directions:

1. Follow the directions given on the package of quinoa and cook the quinoa.
2. Once it is cooked, turn off the heat and fluff the grains using a fork.
3. Meanwhile, make the dressing by adding all the dressing ingredients into a small jar. Fasten the lid and shake the jar to mix well.
4. Place edamame, cucumber, carrot, onion, chickpeas, bell pepper, cherry tomatoes, and parsley in a bowl. Toss well. Pour dressing on top and mix well.
5. To make salad: Place quinoa and vegetable mixture in a bowl and mix well. You can serve it right away or chill and serve later.

57. Mango Avocado Salad

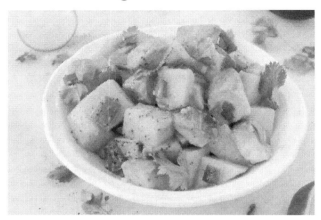

Nutritional values:

- Calories: 312
- Fat: 20 g
- Carbohydrate: 35 g
- Protein: 5.2 g

Ingredients:

- 1 small onion, finely chopped
- ½ avocado, peeled, pitted, cut into cubes
- ¼ cup halved grape tomatoes
- 1 small clove garlic, peeled, minced
- ¼ ripe mango, peeled, cut into cubes
- ½ cucumber, peeled, chopped
- 1 teaspoon fresh lemon juice
- Chopped parsley to garnish

Directions:

1. Combine mango, avocado, cucumber, onion, tomato, garlic, lemon juice, and parsley in a bowl and toss well.
2. You can serve it immediately or chill and serve later.

58. Crispy Sesame Tofu with Zucchini Noodle

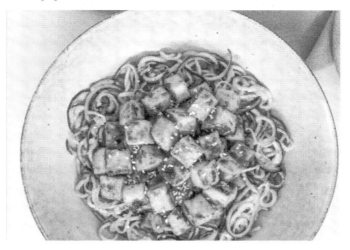

Nutritional values:

- Calories: 397
- Fat: 31 g
- Carbohydrate: 16 g
- Protein: 18 g

Ingredients:

For sesame peanut sauce:

- 2 tablespoons peanut butter
- 1 tablespoon light soy sauce
- ¼ teaspoon chili flakes
- 1 clove garlic, peeled, roughly chopped
- ½ tablespoon sesame oil
- 1 tablespoon rice vinegar
- ½ tablespoon maple syrup or honey
- ¼ teaspoon peeled, grated ginger

For the tofu:

- ¾ teaspoon oil
- ½ small zucchini
- 3 ounces firm tofu, cut into small cubes
- ½ teaspoon sesame seeds, to garnish
- 1 tablespoon thinly sliced green onion to garnish

Directions:

1. To make sesame peanut sauce: Place all the sauce ingredients in a blender and blend until smooth.
2. Pour oil into a pan and let it heat over medium heat. When oil is hot, add tofu and cook until light brown.
3. Pour about a tablespoon of sauce and mix well. Let it cook until golden brown and crisp.
4. Meanwhile, make zucchini noodles using a spiralizer or a julienne peeler.
5. To serve: Place zucchini noodles in a bowl. Pour some of the sauce mixture and toss well.
6. Place tofu on top. Drizzle remaining sauce over the tofu and serve. You can serve this chilled as well but the tofu will not remain crispy.

59. Cauliflower Shawarma Grain Bowl

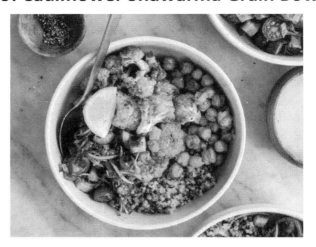

Nutritional values:

- Calories: 505
- Fat: 21 g
- Carbohydrate: 64 g
- Protein: 18 g

Ingredients:

- ¼ cup quinoa
- ¼ can (from a 14.5 ounces can) chickpeas, rinsed, drained
- 2 teaspoons olive oil, divided
- ½ Persian cucumber, cut into ½ inch cubes
- 1 tablespoon chopped parsley
- 1 teaspoon lemon juice
- ¼ teaspoon grated lemon zest
- ¼ head cauliflower, cut into bite size florets
- ½ cup quartered cherry tomatoes
- 1/8 cup thinly sliced onion
- 1 tablespoon chopped mint
- 2 tablespoons tahini dressing

For shawarma spice blend:

- ½ teaspoon cracked black pepper
- ½ teaspoon paprika
- ½ teaspoon cumin
- 1/8 teaspoon turmeric powder
- A pinch garlic powder
- ¼ teaspoon kosher salt
- 1/8 teaspoon red pepper flakes

Directions:

1. The first thing to do is to preheat your oven to 400 °F.

2. Follow the directions given on the package of quinoa and cook the quinoa.

3. Once it is cooked, turn off the heat and fluff the grains using a fork.

4. To make shawarma spice blend, combine all the spices and salt in a bowl.

5. Place cauliflower on one half a baking sheet. Drizzle half the oil over it and sprinkle half the shawarma spice blend and toss well. Spread it evenly.

6. Place chickpeas on the other side of the baking sheet. Drizzle remaining oil and toss well. Spread it evenly.

7. Put the baking sheet into the oven and set the timer for about 25 minutes or until the cauliflower is golden brown and chickpeas are crisp. Whichever cooks first, take it out.

8. When you take out the chickpeas, sprinkle remaining spice mixture over the chickpeas and toss well. When you take out the cauliflower, drizzle lemon juice over it and toss well.

9. To make salad: Combine tomatoes, onion, cucumber, salt, pepper, and herbs in a bowl and toss well.

10. To assemble the bowl, place quinoa in a bowl. Place chickpeas, cauliflower, and tomato salad over the quinoa. Drizzle tahini dressing on top and serve.

60. Creamy Spinach and Feta Cheese Tortilla Wraps

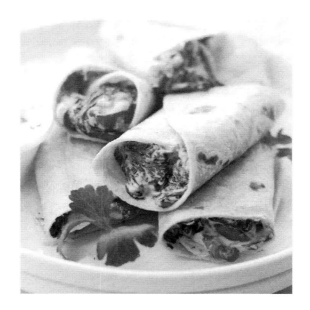

Nutritional values:

- Calories: 287

- Fat: 15 g

- Carbohydrate: 28 g

- Protein: 8 g

Ingredients:

- 2 tablespoons light whipped cream cheese

- ¼ small onion, diced

- Salt to taste

- 2 ounces baby spinach leaves

- ½ green onion, thinly sliced

- 1 tablespoon crumbled feta cheese

- Cooking spray

- ½ tablespoon extra-virgin olive oil

- 1/8 cup thinly sliced red bell pepper

- ½ clove garlic, finely chopped

- Salt to taste

- Freshly ground pepper to taste

- 1 tablespoon shredded parmesan cheese

- 1 whole-wheat tortilla or gluten free tortilla (8 inches)

Directions:

1. The first thing to do is to preheat your oven to 350 °F.

2. Prepare a baking sheet by greasing it with cooking spray.

3. Add cream cheese into a bowl and keep it aside.

4. Pour oil into a skillet and let it heat over medium heat. When oil is hot, add onion and bell pepper and cook for a couple of minutes. Add salt and stir. Cook for another minute or two.

5. Add garlic and cook for a few seconds, until you get a nice aroma.

6. Stir in spinach. Add salt and pepper to taste and cook until spinach turns limp. Turn off the heat. Transfer the spinach mixture into the bowl of cream cheese.

7. Stir in parmesan cheese, green onion and feta cheese and mix well.

8. Spread the mixture on a tortilla. Roll it up and place it in the baking dish. Spray the wrap with cooking spray.

9. Place it in the oven and bake until the tortilla is light brown.

10. Cut into two halves if desired and serve.

61. Coconut Red Curry with Chickpeas

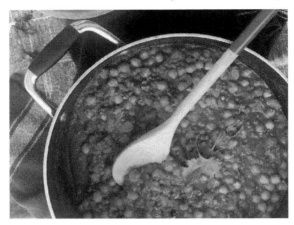

Nutritional values:

- Calories: 343

- Fat: 17.6 g

- Carbohydrate: 40.2 g

- Protein: 12.4 g

Ingredients:

- ¾ teaspoon coconut oil

- 1 large clove garlic, peeled, minced

- ½ dried red chili (optional)

- ¼ medium red bell pepper, chopped

- ½ can (from a 14 ounces can) light coconut milk

- ¼ teaspoon turmeric powder

- ¼ can (from a 15 ounces can) chickpeas, drained, rinsed

- Chopped basil or cilantro to garnish

- ½ medium shallot, minced

- 2–3 teaspoons green or red curry paste

- ¼ cup chopped eggplant

- ¼ can (from a 8 ounces can) bamboo shoots, rinsed, drained

- ½ tablespoon coconut sugar or more to taste

- ¼ cup green peas

- ½ tablespoon minced ginger

- Salt to taste

Directions:

1. Add oil into a small pan and let it melt. When oil melts, add shallot, ginger, and garlic and cook for a few minutes until a bit soft.

2. Stir in curry paste, turmeric, and dried chili. Keep stirring for about a minute.

3. Stir in bell pepper and eggplant. Once it is well combined, add bamboo shoots, coconut milk, salt, chickpea, and coconut sugar. Mix well.

4. Turn down the heat to low heat and cook for about 10 minutes.

5. Stir in peas and cook for a few minutes, until peas are cooked.

6. Sprinkle basil on top and serve it as it is or over rice or noodles or cauliflower rice. The nutritional ingredients of the serving options are not included.

62. Roasted Veggies and Lentils Bowl

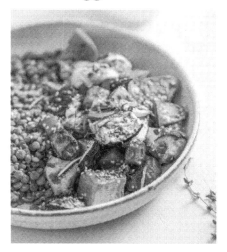

Nutritional values:

- Calories: 288
- Fat: 3.5 g
- Carbohydrate: 56 g
- Protein: 12 g

Ingredients:

- ½ small onion, diced
- ½ medium zucchini, cut into cubes
- ½ teaspoon olive oil
- ½ teaspoon minced fresh thyme or ¼ teaspoon dried thyme
- ½ cup water or vegetable broth
- ½ tablespoon honey
- Pepper to taste
- ½ cup cubed carrot
- ½ medium sweet potato, peeled or scrubbed, cut into cubes
- ½ teaspoon minced fresh rosemary or ¼ teaspoon dried rosemary
- ¼ cup uncooked lentils, rinsed
- ½ tablespoon balsamic vinegar
- Salt to taste

Directions:

1. Set the temperature of your oven to 425 °F and preheat the oven.

2. If you have time on hand, soak the lentils in water for about 40 to 60 minutes. It will cook faster.

3. Toss together carrot, onion, sweet potato, and zucchini in a bowl. Pour oil and toss well. Sprinkle salt and pepper to taste and stir until well combined.

4. Transfer the vegetables onto a baking sheet. Spread the vegetables evenly on the baking sheet. Scatter the herbs over the vegetables.

5. Place the baking sheet in the oven and set the timer for 30 to 40 minutes or until the vegetables are cooked.

6. Boil the broth in a pot. Add lentils and turn down the heat. Cook covered until lentils are cooked.

7. If there is extra broth left in the pot, you can drain it off or leave it as it is.

8. Place lentils, carrot, onion, sweet potato, and zucchini in a bowl. Mix well. Drizzle honey and vinegar on top. Toss well.

9. Serve. You can serve it as it is or over cooked grains of your choice to increase the calorie intake. You can also serve it with bread. The nutritional value of the cooked grains is not included.

63. Spicy Tomatoes and Spinach Pasta

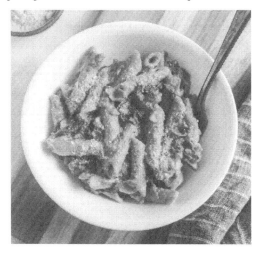

Nutritional values:

- Calories: 524
- Fat: 11 g
- Carbohydrate: 75 g
- Protein: 24 g

Ingredients:

- 1 teaspoon olive oil
- 1 clove garlic, crushed
- 3.5 ounces whole-wheat penne pasta
- ¼ cup red wine
- 2.5 ounces baby spinach
- ½ onion, finely chopped
- ¼ teaspoon dried red chili flakes
- ½ can (from a 14.1 ounces can) chopped tomatoes
- ¼ teaspoon dried oregano
- 2 tablespoons grated parmesan cheese or any other cheese of your choice

Directions:

1. Follow the directions given on the package of pasta and cook the pasta.
2. Pour oil into a pan and let it heat over medium heat. When oil is hot, add onion and garlic and cook until onion turns translucent.
3. Stir in chili flakes. Cook for a few seconds and stir in the tomatoes, oregano, and wine.
4. Turn down the heat to low heat and simmer for about 7–8 minutes. Stir occasionally.
5. Add spinach and mix well. Cook for a couple of minutes, until spinach wilts slightly.
6. Add pasta and toss well.
7. Transfer the pasta into a bowl. Scatter cheese on top and serve.

64. Black Bean Quesadillas

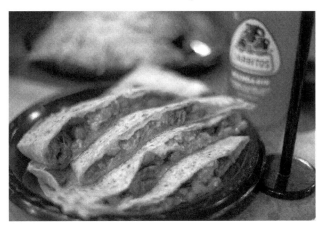

Nutritional values:

- Calories: 375
- Fat: 16 g
- Carbohydrate: 45 g
- Protein: 13 g

Ingredients:

- ¼ can (from a 15 ounces can) black beans, rinsed, drained
- 2 tablespoons prepared fresh salsa, divided
- ½ teaspoon canola oil
- ¼ cup shredded Monterey Pepper Jack cheese
- 1 whole-wheat tortillas (8 inches)
- ½ ripe avocado, peeled, pitted, diced

Directions:

1. Add beans, 1 tablespoon salsa, and cheese into a bowl. Mix well.

2. Place the tortilla on a plate. Spread the bean filling over one half of the tortilla. Fold the other half of the tortilla over the filling. Press gently.

3. Place a nonstick skillet over medium heat. Add oil and swirl the pan to spread the oil.

4. Place the quesadilla in the pan. Cook until the underside is golden brown. Turn the quesadilla over and cook the other side until golden brown.

5. Remove the quesadilla from the pan and place on a plate. Cut into two halves if desired.

6. Drizzle remaining salsa on top and serve with avocado.

65. Flatbread Pizza

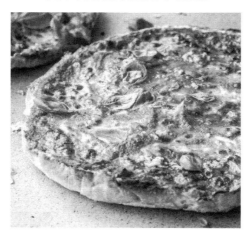

Nutritional values:

- Calories: 442
- Fat: 24.9 g
- Carbohydrate: 38.2 g
- Protein: 17.7 g

Ingredients:

- 1 flatbread (about 6–8 inches diameter)
- 2 ounces fresh mozzarella cheese, sliced
- ½ large tomato, cut into thin, round slices
- ¼ teaspoon dried oregano
- ½ tablespoon extra-virgin olive oil + extra to serve
- 4 fresh basil leaves + extra to garnish
- Salt to taste
- Freshly ground black pepper to taste
- 1 small clove garlic, peeled, minced

Directions:

1. Set the temperature of your oven to 425 °F and preheat the oven.
2. Prepare a baking sheet by lining it with parchment paper.
3. Combine oil and garlic in a small bowl. Let it infuse for 10 minutes.
4. Brush oil over the flatbread. Place mozzarella cheese slices over the flatbread. Scatter basil leaves. Place tomato slices over the cheese.
5. Sprinkle a generous amount of salt and pepper. Sprinkle oregano as well.
6. Place the baking sheet in the oven and set the timer for 10–15 minutes or until the cheese melts and is browned at a few spots.
7. Cut into wedges. Drizzle some oil on top.
8. Scatter some basil leaves on top and serve.

66. Green Goddess Salad with Chickpeas

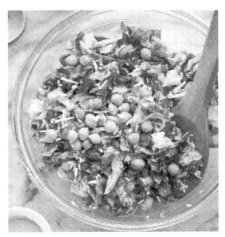

Nutritional values:

- Calories: 304
- Fat: 7.5 g
- Carbohydrate: 39.8 g
- Protein: 21.7 g

Ingredients:

For the dressing:

- ½ avocado, peeled, pitted, chopped
- 1/8 cup chopped fresh herbs of your choice
- Salt to taste
- ¾ cup buttermilk
- 1 tablespoon rice vinegar

For salad:

- 1 ½ cups chopped romaine lettuce
- ½ can (from a 15 ounces can) chickpeas, rinsed
- 3 cherry tomatoes, halved
- ½ cup sliced cucumber

- 1/8 cup diced low-fat Swiss cheese

Directions:

1. If you do not have buttermilk, you can make it at home by combining ¾ cup milk (at room temperature) with 2 teaspoons lemon juice or vinegar. Once it is combined, let it rest for about 10 minutes. You will notice some curdling of milk. The buttermilk is now ready.
2. To make dressing: Add buttermilk, avocado, vinegar, herbs, and salt into a blender. Blend until you get a smooth mixture.
3. To make salad: Combine cucumber and lettuce in a bowl. Add about 2 tablespoons of the dressing and mix well. Taste the salad and add more dressing if desired.
4. Transfer the salad into a serving bowl. Scatter cheese, chickpeas, and tomatoes on top.
5. Serve.
6. The remaining dressing can be saved in an airtight container in the refrigerator for about 3 days.

67. Spiced Cauliflower and Chickpea Salad

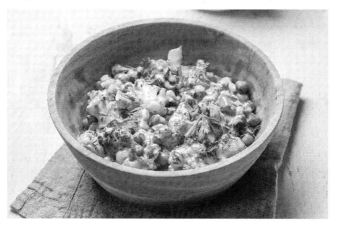

Nutritional values:

- Calories: 241
- Fat: 9.4 g
- Carbohydrate: 32.6 g
- Protein: 10.6 g

Ingredients:

For the salad:

- ½ tablespoon curry powder
- Salt to taste
- ½ cup cooked or canned chickpeas, rinsed, drained
- ½ tablespoon olive oil
- ¾ cup cauliflower florets
- 1 small carrot, cut into ½ inch thick slices

- 1 cup torn lettuce leaves
- 1/8 cup thinly sliced red onion
- ½ cup packed fresh Italian parsley

For the dressing:

- 1/8 cup low-fat plain yogurt
- Pepper to taste
- ½ tablespoon lime juice
- ¼ teaspoon grated fresh ginger
- ½ tablespoon fat-free milk (optional)
- ¼ teaspoon minced jalapeño pepper

Directions:

1. Set the temperature of your oven to 450 °F and preheat the oven.

2. Combine chickpeas, cauliflower, and carrots in a bowl.

3. Drizzle oil over the mixture and toss well. Sprinkle salt and curry powder and toss well.

4. Transfer the mixture into a baking dish and spread it evenly. Place the baking dish in the oven and set the timer for about 30 minutes. Keep a watch over the ingredients in the oven after about 20 minutes of roasting.

5. Stir the mixture every 15 minutes.

6. In the meantime, make the dressing by whisking together ginger, lime juice, yogurt, and jalapeño in a bowl. Add milk if using and whisk well.

7. To make salad: Place roasted carrot, cauliflower, and chickpeas in a bowl and toss well.

8. Add lettuce, onion, and parsley and toss well.

9. Pour dressing on top and toss well and serve.

68. Black Bean Salad

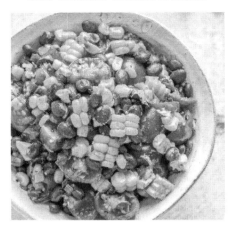

Nutritional values:

- Calories: 322
- Fat: 16 g
- Carbohydrate: 40.8 g
- Protein: 10.6 g

Ingredients:

For the dressing:

- 1 tablespoon chopped cilantro
- ¼ medium ripe avocado, pitted, roughly chopped
- 1 tablespoon lime juice
- Salt to taste
- ½ clove garlic, peeled, minced
- ½ tablespoon extra-virgin olive oil

For the salad:

- ¼ cup thinly sliced red onion
- ½ cup frozen corn kernels
- ¼ can (from a 15 ounces can) black beans, drained, rinsed
- 2 cups mixed salad greens
- ½ cup halved grape tomatoes

Directions:

1. Add onions into a bowl of cold water and keep it aside.
2. Place cilantro, avocado, oil, lime juice, salt, and garlic into a small blender and blend until very smooth.
3. Add corn, greens, beans, and tomatoes into a bowl and toss well.
4. Remove the onions from the bowl of water and add them into the salad bowl. Toss well.
5. Pour dressing over the salad. Mix well and serve.

Snack Recipes

Forget about chips and biscuits, because these aren't the only snacking options available. In this section, you will be introduced to several macro diet-friendly snack recipes. Whether you want to fill a nutritional gap in your daily nutrition or need to increase your calorie and macros intake, these recipes will come in handy.

69. Baked Spicy Chicken Wings

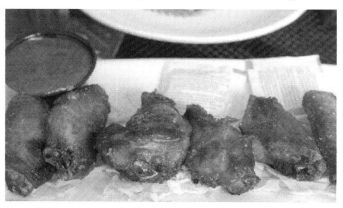

Nutritional values:

- Calories: 176

- Fat: 15 g

- Carbohydrate: 1.5 g

- Protein: 9 g

Ingredients:

- 4 ounces chicken wings

- ½ teaspoon paprika or to taste

- Salt to taste

- ½ teaspoon avocado oil

- 1 ½ tablespoons hot sauce

- ¼ teaspoon garlic powder

- ¼ teaspoon dried oregano

- 1/8 teaspoon red chili flakes

- ½ teaspoon apple cider vinegar

- Cooking spray

Directions:

1. Firstly preheat your oven to 350 °F. Prepare a baking sheet by lining it with foil. Grease it with cooking spray.

2. Combine salt and all the spices in a bowl. Sprinkle this mixture over the chicken wings and rub it into the wings.

3. Place the wings on the baking sheet and put it into the oven. Set the timer for about 30 minutes or bake until crisp.

4. Add oil, hot sauce, garlic powder, salt if required, and vinegar into a small saucepan. Place it over low heat.

5. Stir often for about 3 minutes. Turn off the heat. Place chicken in a bowl. Drizzle the sauce mixture over the chicken. Mix well and serve.

70. Coconut Pineapple Shrimp Skewers

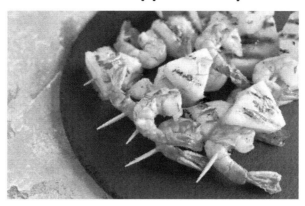

Nutritional values:

- Calories: 165
- Fat: 2 g
- Carbohydrate: 12 g
- Protein: 24 g

Ingredients:

- 1/8 cup light coconut milk
- ½ teaspoon soy sauce
- 1 tablespoon fresh lime juice
- 3 ounces pineapple, cut into 1 inch pieces
- Chopped cilantro to garnish
- Sliced green onion to garnish
- 1 teaspoon tabasco red sauce or any other hot sauce
- 1 tablespoon fresh orange juice
- 4 ounces large shrimp
- Oil to grill

Directions:

1. Add tabasco sauce, coconut milk, orange juice, soy sauce, and lime juice into a bowl and whisk well.
2. Drop the shrimp into the bowl and stir until shrimp is well coated with the mixture.
3. Cover the bowl and chill for a couple of hours. Make sure to stir the mixture every 30 to 40 minutes.
4. In case you want to use wooden skewers, make sure to soak them in water for about 30 minutes before grilling.
5. Set up your grill and preheat it to medium-high heat. Take out the shrimp from the bowl and thread it onto one to two skewers. Do not discard the marinade.
6. Put the pineapple pieces in between the shrimp. Place the skewer on the grill and let it grill for about 3 minutes. Turn every minute. Brush with marinade while grilling.
7. Once the shrimp are grilled, transfer onto a serving plate. Garnish with cilantro and green onion and serve.

71. Rainbow Collard Wraps with Peanut Butter Dipping Sauce

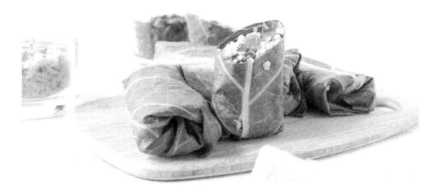

Nutritional values:

- Calories: 264 + 212 = 476
- Fat: 18 g + 17 g = 35 g
- Carbohydrate: 25 g + 10 g = 35 g
- Protein: 7 g + 8 g = 15 g

Ingredients:

For the wrap:

- 1 large collard green leaf
- 1 carrot, julienne cut
- ½ avocado, peeled, pitted, cut into thick slices
- 1/8 cup basil leaves
- 1/8 cup hummus
- ¼ English cucumber, julienne cut
- 1/8 red cabbage, shredded
- 1/8 cup mint leaves

For dipping sauce:

- 2 tablespoons peanut butter
- ½ tablespoon soy sauce or tamari
- ¼ teaspoon garlic powder
- ½ tablespoon sweet chili sauce
- 1 tablespoon rice vinegar

Directions:

1. Put the collard leaf in a pot of boiling water for about 30 seconds. Remove it and place it over paper towels. Pat the top of the leaf with paper towels until dry.

2. Carefully slice the thick part of the stem so that you can roll it up.

3. Smear hummus on the leaf. Place carrot, avocado, cucumber, cabbage, mint, and basil along the length of the leaf at the center.

4. Fold like a burrito. Cut into two halves if desired before serving.

5. To make dipping sauce, combine all the dipping sauce ingredients in a bowl.

6. Serve wrap with dipping sauce right away.

72. Crispy Parmesan Garlic Edamame

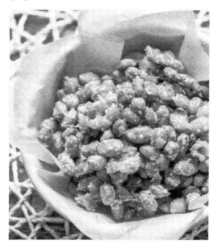

Nutritional values:

- Calories: 150
- Fat: 9 g
- Carbohydrate: 8 g
- Protein: 10 g

Ingredients:

- ½ cup edamame, uncooked
- 1 tablespoon grated parmesan cheese
- Salt to taste
- ¾ teaspoon olive oil
- A pinch garlic powder
- Black pepper to taste

Directions:

1. Firstly preheat your oven to 350 °F. Prepare a baking sheet by lining it with parchment paper.

2. Combine garlic powder, pepper, parmesan, and salt in a bowl.

3. Thaw the edamame if frozen and place in a bowl. Drizzle oil over the edamame and toss well.

4. Sprinkle the parmesan mixture over the edamame and toss well.

5. Transfer the edamame onto the prepared baking sheet and spread it evenly.

6. Place the baking sheet in the oven and set the timer for about 12 to 15 minutes, depending on how you like it cooked.

7. Take out the baking sheet from the oven and let it rest for 5 to 8 minutes.

8. Serve.

73. Devilled Eggs

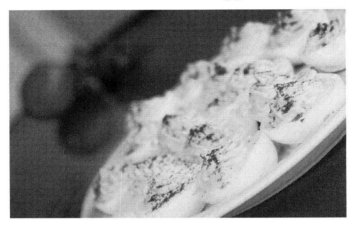

Nutritional values:

- Calories: 127
- Fat: 11 g
- Carbohydrate: 1 g
- Protein: 7 g

Ingredients:

- 1 egg, hardboiled, peeled, halved lengthwise
- ¼ teaspoon chopped parsley
- Salt to taste
- Paprika to garnish
- A pinch ground mustard
- ½ teaspoon chia seeds
- 1 ½ teaspoons mayonnaise

Directions:

1. Carefully remove the yolk from the egg halves and place in a bowl.
2. Add mayonnaise, parsley, chia seeds, mustard and salt and mix well.
3. Fill this mixture in the cavity of the egg whites.
4. Sprinkle paprika on top. Chill for an hour and serve. You can eat 2 to 3 eggs to fulfill your calorie intake.

74. Rosemary Roasted Almonds

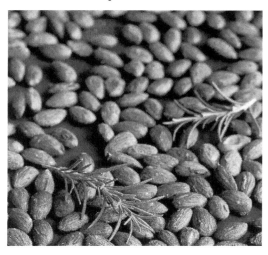

Nutritional values:

- Calories: 222

- Fat: 19.8 g

- Carbohydrate: 7.2 g

- Protein: 7.6 g

Ingredients:

- ½ teaspoon finely chopped fresh rosemary

- 1/8 teaspoon chili powder or to taste

- Ground red pepper to taste

- ½ teaspoon extra-virgin olive oil

- Salt to taste

- ¼ cup whole almonds

Directions:

1. Set the temperature of your oven to 325 °F and preheat the oven. Prepare a baking sheet by lining it with foil.

2. Place almonds in a bowl. Drizzle oil over the almonds. Sprinkle chili powder, pepper, salt, and rosemary and toss well.

3. Spread the almonds on the baking sheet. Place the baking sheet in the oven and set the timer for 8–10 minutes or until toasted lightly. Keep a watch over the almonds as they can get burnt.

4. Let the almonds cool completely. Serve.

5. You can make 4–5 servings and place them in an airtight container. It is a very handy and healthy snack.

75. Bruschetta

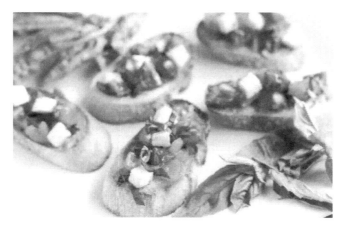

Nutritional values:

- Calories: 144
- Fat: 4.3 g
- Carbohydrate: 20.1 g
- Protein: 6.6 g

Ingredients:

- 1/8 cup quartered cherry tomatoes
- ½ tablespoon grated parmesan cheese
- 1 teaspoon Italian dressing
- ½ clove garlic, peeled
- Freshly ground pepper to taste
- Salt to taste
- 1 tablespoon shredded mozzarella cheese
- ½ tablespoon chopped basil
- 1 slice French bread (about ¼ inch thick)

Directions:

1. Set the oven to broil mode and preheat the oven.
2. Toast the bread slice lightly. Rub garlic over the bread slice.
3. Add tomatoes, basil, parmesan cheese, mozzarella cheese, salt, pepper, and Italian dressing into a bowl and mix well.
4. Spread the mixture over the toasted bread slice.
5. Place bruschetta on a baking sheet and put the baking sheet in the oven. Broil for a couple of minutes until the cheese melts.
6. Take out the bruschetta from the oven and cool for a couple of minutes before serving.

76. Potato Soup

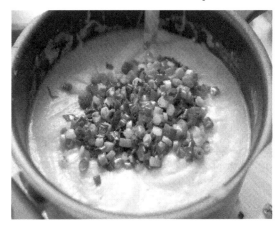

Nutritional values:

- Calories: 460
- Fat: 12.1 g
- Carbohydrate: 72 g
- Protein: 18.4 g

Ingredients:

- ¾ pound russet potatoes, peeled, cut into 1 inch cubes
- ¼ cup shredded cheddar cheese
- ¼ teaspoon garlic powder
- ½ cup 2% milk
- 3 green onions, chopped (use only the greens)
- Black pepper to taste
- ¼ teaspoon salt or to taste

Directions:

1. Place potatoes in a pot. Pour enough water to cover the potatoes with water. Place the pot over medium heat.

2. When it begins to boil, lower the heat and simmer until potatoes are soft and almost breaking off.

3. Retain some of the cooked water in the pot itself and drain off the rest, depending on the consistency of the soup you desire.

4. Stir in garlic powder, milk, salt, and pepper.

5. Mash the potatoes with a fork until the texture you desire is achieved. You can leave it chunky or make it smooth.

6. Place the pot over low heat. Simmer for 3–4 minutes.

7. Ladle the soup into a soup bowl.

8. Sprinkle green onions and cheese on top. Season with salt and pepper and serve.

Side Dish

A side dish can quickly elevate the overall feel of any meal. Whether it's a portion of roasted vegetables or a healthy mash, there are plenty of options to choose from. While making a meal plan, if you have any additional calorie quota to fulfill, these recipes will help!

77. Healthy Mashed Sweet Potatoes

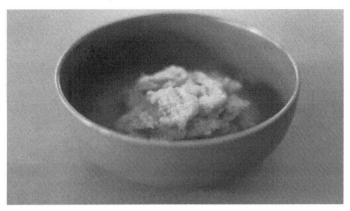

Nutritional values:

- Calories: 130
- Fat: 3 g
- Carbohydrate: 24 g
- Protein: 2 g

Ingredients:

- 4 ounces sweet potatoes, peeled, chopped into chunks
- 1 tablespoon low-fat milk
- Pepper to taste
- ½ teaspoon minced fresh thyme, to garnish
- ¾ teaspoon butter
- Kosher salt to taste
- A pinch ground cinnamon

Directions:

1. Cook sweet potato in a small pot of boiling water until fork tender.

2. Drain off the water from the pot and add salt, cinnamon, butter, and milk. Mash up the ingredients together using a potato masher.

3. Sprinkle thyme on top and serve.

78. Roasted Vegetables

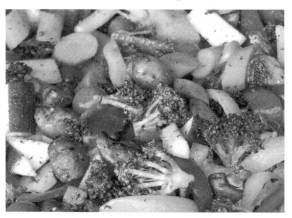

Nutritional values:

- Calories: 199
- Fat: 11 g
- Carbohydrate: 23 g
- Protein: 5 g

Ingredients:

- 1.5 ounces baby potatoes, halved
- 1.5 ounces bell pepper, diced
- 1.5 ounces grape tomatoes
- 1.5 ounces broccoli florets
- 1 ounce baby carrots
- 1 ounce zucchini, sliced
- 1 ounce onion, diced
- ¼ teaspoon chopped fresh thyme
- ¾ tablespoon olive oil
- 3 cloves garlic, peeled
- Chopped fresh parsley to garnish
- Salt to taste
- Pepper to taste
- 1 teaspoon grated parmesan cheese

Directions:

1. Firstly preheat your oven to 400 °F.
2. Place potatoes, garlic, bell pepper, tomatoes, broccoli, carrots, zucchini, onion, thyme, salt, pepper, and oregano in a bowl and toss well.
3. Add oil and mix well.
4. Remove potatoes, garlic, and carrots from the bowl and place it on a baking sheet.
5. Place the baking sheet in the oven and set the timer for 10 minutes.
6. Now add the rest of the vegetables and continue baking for 10–15 minutes or until vegetables are cooked through.
7. Transfer the roasted vegetables into a bowl. Garnish with parmesan cheese and parsley and serve.

79. Roasted Brussels Sprouts

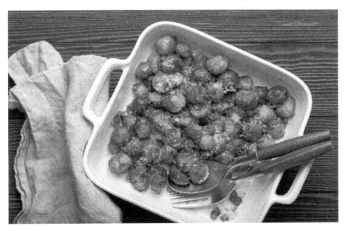

Nutritional values:

- Calories: 104

- Fat: 7.3 g

- Carbohydrate: 10 g

- Protein: 2.9 g

Ingredients:

- 6 ounces Brussels sprouts, trimmed, discard yellow leaves

- Salt to taste

- ¾ tablespoon olive oil

- Freshly ground pepper to taste

Directions:

1. Start off by preheating your oven to 400 °F.

2. Place Brussels sprouts in a bowl. Sprinkle salt and pepper over them. Drizzle oil and mix well.

3. Spread on a baking sheet and put it into the oven. Set the timer for about 30 minutes or until brown. Make sure to turn the Brussels sprouts every 5 to 6 minutes so that they are browned evenly.

4. The roasted Brussels sprouts should be dark brown in color.

5. Serve hot.

80. Sautéed Broccoli Stir Fry Recipe with Garlic

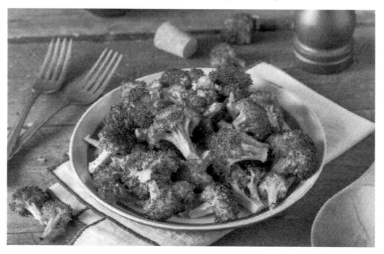

Nutritional values:

- Calories: 148
- Fat: 14 g
- Carbohydrate: 6 g
- Protein: 2 g

Ingredients:

- 1 tablespoon olive oil
- 1 cup broccoli florets
- Pepper to taste
- 1 clove garlic, minced
- Salt to taste
- 1 tablespoon water

Directions:

1. Pour oil into a pan and place it over medium heat. When oil is hot, add garlic and cook for a few seconds until you get a nice aroma.

2. Stir in broccoli, salt, and pepper. Raise the heat to medium-high heat.

3. Cook for a few minutes, stirring often until they turn bright green in color and slightly brown as well.

4. Drizzle water and cover the pan. Cook for a couple of minutes. Uncover and cook until dry.

5. Serve hot.

81. Stuffed Delicata Squash

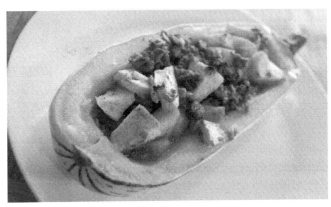

Nutritional values:

- Calories: 282
- Fat: 11.2 g
- Carbohydrate: 44.5 g
- Protein: 6.5 g

Ingredients:

- ½ delicata squash, deseeded
- 1 apple, peeled, cored, diced
- 2 small cloves garlic, minced
- A pinch ground cinnamon
- 1 slice bacon, cooked, crumbled
- 1 teaspoon olive oil or more if required, divided
- 1/8 cup diced onion
- ¼ teaspoon finely chopped fresh rosemary
- Salt to taste
- Freshly ground pepper to taste

Directions:

1. Make sure you cut the squash lengthwise when you cut the whole squash.
2. Set the temperature of your oven to 400 °F and preheat the oven.
3. Brush half the oil inside and cut part of the squash. Keep it on a baking sheet. Place the baking sheet in the oven and set the timer for 30 minutes or bake until fork tender.
4. Pour remaining oil into a skillet and let it heat over medium heat. When oil is hot, add onion and apple and cook until onion is pink.
5. Add rosemary, garlic, and cinnamon and stir. Add salt and pepper to taste.
6. Turn down the heat to low heat and cook until the apple is tender.
7. Stuff the apple mixture into the squash. Scatter bacon on top and serve.
8. You can use any other squash instead of delicata squash like summer squash, etc.

82. Sesame Green Beans

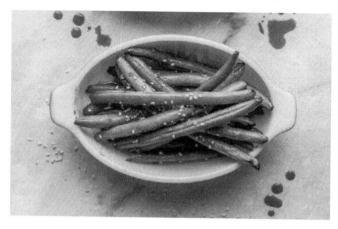

Nutritional values:

- Calories: 196

- Fat: 16.5 g

- Carbohydrate: 8.7 g

- Protein: 3.8 g

Ingredients:

- 1 tablespoon olive oil

- 4 ounces frozen green beans, thawed

- ¼ teaspoon Hickory smoked salt or regular salt

- ½ tablespoon sesame seeds

- ½ tablespoon bacon bits (optional)

- A pinch garlic powder

- Red pepper flakes to taste

Directions:

1. Pour oil into a pan and let it heat over medium heat. When oil is hot, add sesame seeds and keep stirring until it is lightly toasted. Be careful as it can burn.

2. Stir in green beans, salt, bacon bits if using, and garlic powder.

3. Stir-fry for 2 to 3 minutes. Add red pepper flakes and stir. Turn off the heat.

4. Serve hot.

83. Eggplant Parmesan

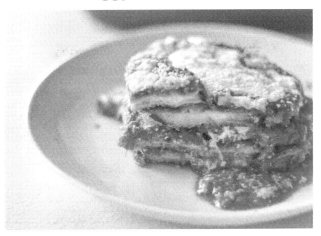

Nutritional values:

- Calories: 275
- Fat: 21 g
- Carbohydrate: 16 g
- Protein: 9 g

Ingredients:

- 1 tablespoon olive oil
- ½ small eggplant, peeled, cut into ½ inch thick, round slices
- ½ tablespoon grated parmesan cheese
- ¼ cup shredded mozzarella cheese
- ½ clove garlic, minced
- Salt to taste
- ½ tablespoon minced fresh basil or ½ teaspoon dried basil + extra to garnish
- ½ medium tomato, cut into thin, round slices
- Pepper to taste

Directions:

1. Set the temperature of your oven to 425 °F and preheat the oven.
2. Prepare a baking dish by greasing it with some cooking spray.
3. Mix together oil and garlic in a small bowl and brush it over the eggplant slices, on either side.
4. Place the eggplant slices in the baking dish. Set the timer for 20 minutes. Turn the eggplant slices over after 15 minutes of baking.
5. Set aside half the eggplant slices on a plate. Scatter half the basil and parmesan cheese on half the eggplant slices that are remaining in the baking dish. Place tomato slices over these eggplant slices. Scatter remaining basil and parmesan over the tomatoes.
6. Spread half the mozzarella cheese over the tomatoes. Now place remaining eggplant slices over these. Place remaining mozzarella cheese on top. Cover the baking dish with foil and put it in the oven. Set the timer for 25 minutes.
7. Uncover after about 20 minutes and bake for the remaining 5 minutes.
8. Cool for 5 minutes and serve.

84. Vegetables Stuffed Tomatoes

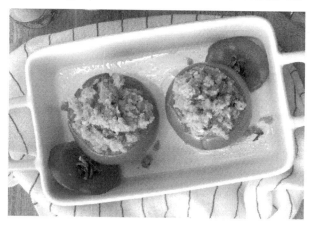

Nutritional values:

- Calories: 182
- Fat: 7 g
- Carbohydrate: 23 g
- Protein: 6 g

Ingredients:

- 1 medium tomato
- ¼ celery rib, sliced
- ½ small clove garlic, peeled
- 1 teaspoon olive oil
- 3 tablespoons dry breadcrumbs
- 2 fresh basil leaves, thinly sliced
- ¼ small carrot, peeled, chopped
- ¼ small onion
- 1/8 teaspoon dried oregano
- ½ tablespoon white wine or vegetable broth
- 1 tablespoon grated parmesan cheese
- Salt to taste
- Pepper to taste

Directions:

1. Take a sharp knife and cut a thin slice from the stem part of the tomato. With a spoon, carefully remove the pulp of the tomato and keep it aside.
2. Place layers of paper towels on a plate. Place the tomato on the paper towels, with the cut part on the paper towels. Let it remain this way for 5 to 8 minutes.
3. Place onion, celery, garlic, carrot, and tomato pulp in the food processor bowl and process until finely chopped.
4. Pour oil into a pan and let it heat over medium heat. When oil is hot, add the chopped vegetables and oregano and cook until the vegetables are slightly tender.
5. Stir in wine and cook until the liquid in the pan is half its original quantity. Turn off the heat and let it cool for a few minutes.
6. Add breadcrumbs, basil, and parmesan cheese and mix well. Add salt and pepper to taste and turn off the heat.
7. Fill this mixture into the tomato. Keep it in a greased baking dish and put the baking dish in the oven.
8. Bake for 15–20 minutes.
9. Serve.

Dessert Recipes

Following the macros diet will change your relationship with food for the better! You needn't give up on desserts for the sake of the diet. Instead, it is about shifting to healthier options for your sweet tooth cravings. In fact, if you look at the sample meal plans, one thing that stands out is it makes an allowance for a dessert every day! Indulge in these delicious guilt-free and healthy desserts!

85. Chocolate Chia Pudding

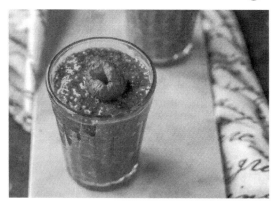

Nutritional values:

- Calories: 517
- Fat: 39 g
- Carbohydrate: 39 g
- Protein: 8.5 g

Ingredients:

- 2 tablespoons chia seeds
- 1 tablespoon cacao powder
- ½ teaspoon vanilla extract
- Few frozen berries to garnish (optional)
- ½ cup coconut milk
- 1 tablespoon maple syrup
- 1 tablespoon dark chocolate chips
- Unsweetened shredded coconut (optional)

Directions:

1. Combine chia seeds, cacao powder, vanilla, milk, chocolate chips, and maple syrup in a glass.

2. Keep the jar covered with cling wrap in the refrigerator for 6–8 hours.

3. Garnish with berries and shredded coconut and serve. The nutritional value of the optional ingredients are not included.

86. Chocolate Orange Protein Ball

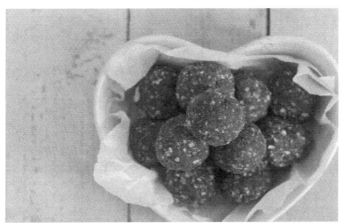

Nutritional values: 3 balls

- Calories: 342

- Fat: 18.3 g

- Carbohydrate: 17.25 g

- Protein: 25.3 g

Ingredients:

- 1 ½ tablespoon almond butter or peanut butter

- 3 teaspoon cocoa powder

- 1 ½ tablespoon almond milk

- 2 ¼ teaspoon grated orange zest

- 2 ¼ teaspoon ground almonds

- 2 ¼ teaspoon maple syrup

- ¾ scoop protein powder

- Melted chocolate (optional)

Directions:

1. Place almond butter, cocoa powder, almond milk, orange zest, ground almonds, maple syrup, and protein powder in a bowl.

2. Mix well using your hand. Shape into a ball. Dip the ball in melted chocolate if desired. Chill for about two hours before serving. The nutritional value of melted chocolate is not included.

87. Chocolate Ice Cream

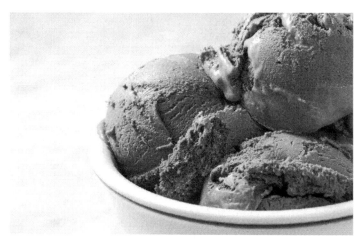

Nutritional values:

- Calories: 180
- Fat: 2.25 g
- Carbohydrate: 4.5 g
- Protein: 12.75 g

Ingredients:

1. 1 ½ cups almond milk
2. 1 ½ tablespoons cocoa powder
3. ¾ teaspoon vanilla extract
4. 1 ½ scoops protein powder
5. 1 ½ packets stevia or stevia drops to taste

Directions:

1. Place milk, cacao powder, vanilla, protein powder, and stevia in a bowl and whisk well.
2. Pour into a small freezer safe container and freeze until firm.
3. Serve.

88. Brownie

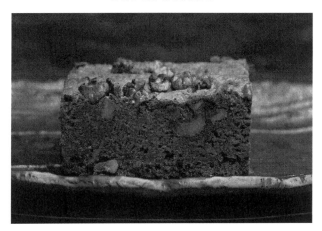

Nutritional values:

- Calories: 125
- Fat: 5 g
- Carbohydrate: 6 g
- Protein: 14 g

Ingredients:

- ½ scoop chocolate protein powder
- 1 tablespoon granulated sweetener of your choice (optional)
- ½–1 tablespoon cocoa powder or cacao powder
- 1/8 cup milk of your choice
- ½ tablespoon coconut flour
- ¼ teaspoon baking powder
- 1 small egg or ½ flax egg or 2 tablespoons egg whites
- ½ tablespoon chocolate chips

Directions:

1. Take a cup or a small bowl and grease it with some cooking spray.
2. Add all the dry ingredients into a small mixing bowl, i.e. coconut flour, protein powder, sweetener, baking powder, and cocoa powder and mix well.
3. Beat egg in a bowl adding milk. Pour it into the mixing bowl and stir until well combined.
4. Pour the batter into the cup or bowl. Scatter chocolate chips on top.
5. Place it in the microwave and cook on high for 50 to 60 seconds.
6. Serve.
7. The nutritional value of the sweetener is not included as your protein powder may have sweetener and if so, you need not add sweetener.

89. Birthday Cake Shake

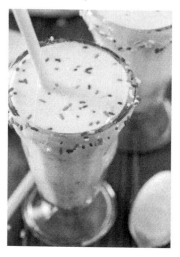

Nutritional values:

- Calories: 165

- Fat: 0.5 g

- Carbohydrate: 23 g

- Protein: 13.5 g

Ingredients:

- ¼ scoop vanilla ice cream flavored whey protein powder

- ¼ cup fat-free milk

- 1 tablespoon Jell-O sugar-free, fat-free vanilla pudding mix

- ½ tablespoon sprinkles

- ¼ medium banana, sliced, frozen

- ¼ cup vanilla flavored non-fat Greek yogurt

- ½ teaspoon vanilla extract

- ½ cup crushed ice

Directions:

1. Place milk, banana, whey protein powder, pudding mix, yogurt, and vanilla in a blender and blend until smooth.

2. Add ice and blend until thick.

3. Pour into a glass and serve.

90. Gluten—Free Protein Lava Cake

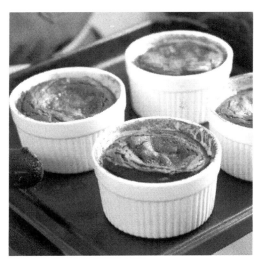

Nutritional values:

- Calories: 295
- Fat: 14.8 g
- Carbohydrate: 27.5 g
- Protein: 20.1 g

Ingredients:

- ½ small chocolate flavored protein bar, chopped into small bite size pieces
- 1 ½ tablespoon dark chocolate chips + extra to garnish
- 1 ½ tablespoons coconut milk or almond milk
- 1 tablespoon oat flour
- 1 tablespoon protein powder
- 1 small egg
- Nonstick cooking spray

Directions:

1. Start off by preheating your oven to 400 °F. Grease a ramekin with cooking spray.
2. Add dark chocolate and milk into a microwave safe bowl and cook for about 30 seconds or until it melts.
3. Combine egg flour and protein powder in a bowl and stir. Add egg and stir until just combined, making sure not to over-mix.
4. Pour the melted chocolate and stir until just combined.
5. Pour half the batter into the ramekin. Scatter protein bar pieces over the batter. Scatter some extra chocolate chips as well.
6. Pour remaining batter into the ramekin. Place it in the oven and set the timer for 10 minutes.
7. Take out the ramekin. Let it cool for 4 to 5 minutes.
8. Serve.

91. Pumpkin and Peanut Butter Cup

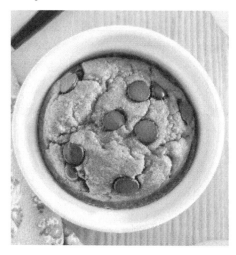

Nutritional values:

- Calories: 173

- Fat: 5 g

- Carbohydrate: 20 g

- Protein: 16 g

Ingredients:

- ¼ cup chocolate protein powder

- 1/8 cup pumpkin puree

- 1 tablespoon honey

- ½ tablespoon mini chocolate chips

- ¼ cup powdered peanut butter

- 1/8 cup egg whites

- 1 tablespoon cocoa powder

- 2 teaspoons creamy peanut butter

Directions:

1. Add protein powder, pumpkin puree, honey, powdered peanut butter, cocoa powder, and egg whites into a bowl and whisk well.

2. Pour into a microwave safe ramekin. Top with peanut butter and chocolate chips.

3. Cook on high in the microwave for a minute.

4. Cool for a few minutes and serve.

92. Eggless Chocolate Mousse

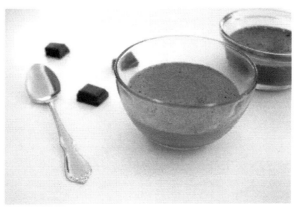

Nutritional values:

- Calories: 127

- Fat: 1.4 g

- Carbohydrate: 22.3 g

- Protein: 7.8 g

Ingredients:

- 4 ounces soft, silken tofu

- 2 tablespoons maple syrup

- ½ tablespoon cocoa powder

- ¼ teaspoon raspberry extract or vanilla extract

Directions:

1. Place tofu, maple syrup, cocoa powder, and raspberry or vanilla extract in a blender and blend until smooth and creamy.

2. Spoon the mixture into a bowl.

3. Chill for 6–8 hours and serve.

93. Black Forest Banana Split

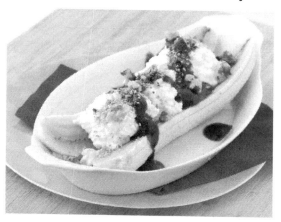

Nutritional values:

- Calories: 377
- Fat: 11 g
- Carbohydrate: 40 g
- Protein: 23 g

Ingredients:

- 1 cup nonfat ricotta cheese
- 8 walnut halves
- 1 teaspoon cherry concentrate or any other fruit concentrate
- 1 banana, peeled, split lengthwise
- ½ teaspoon cocoa powder, unsweetened

Directions:

1. Place ricotta cheese in a dessert bowl. Place a banana half on either side of the cheese in the bowl.

2. Top with walnut halves and sprinkle cocoa powder.

3. Trickle a cherry concentrate on top and serve.

94. Marsala Poached Figs Over Ricotta

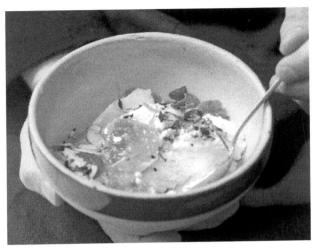

Nutritional values:

- Calories: 228
- Fat: 6.9 g
- Carbohydrate: 37.1 g
- Protein: 9 g

Ingredients:

- ¼ cup quartered dried figs
- 1 teaspoon honey
- ½ teaspoon brown sugar
- ½ tablespoon toasted, slivered almonds
- 2 tablespoons Marsala or port wine
- ¼ cup part-skim ricotta cheese
- 5–6 drops vanilla extract

Directions:

1. Combine figs, honey, and Marsala wine in a small saucepan.

2. Place the saucepan over low heat and stir often until figs are soft and the sauce is thick like syrup. Turn off the heat.

3. Combine sugar, ricotta, and vanilla in a dessert bowl. Spoon the fig mixture on top. Garnish with almond slivers and serve.

95. Summer Berry Pudding

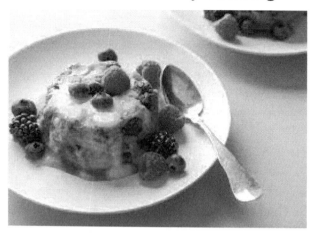

Nutritional values:

- Calories: 243
- Fat: 2.3 g
- Carbohydrate: 54.8 g
- Protein: 4.6 g

Ingredients:

- 2 small slices firm white bread, remove the crusts
- ½ cup fresh blueberries
- ½ cup sliced fresh strawberries
- ½ cup fresh raspberries
- A pinch salt
- 1 tablespoon water
- 1 tablespoon brown sugar

Directions:

1. Place bread slices on your cutting board. Invert a ramekin on the bread and cut the bread into a round. Repeat with the other bread slice.

2. Add berries, water, sugar, and salt into a small saucepan and place it over medium-high heat. Cook for a few minutes until the berries burst and are broken down.

3. Retain a little of the berry mixture to garnish and place it in the refrigerator once it cools.

4. Spoon about a tablespoon of the hot berry mixture into the ramekin. Place a slice of bread inside the ramekin. Pour remaining berry mixture over the bread slice.

5. Keep the other bread slice on top of the berry mixture.

6. Place the ramekin on a plate and cover the ramekin with cling wrap. Place something heavy on top of the pudding like a cold drink can. Chill for 6–8 hours.

7. Take a knife and run it around the inner edges of the ramekin and invert the pudding on a plate.

8. Drizzle the retained berry mixture on top and serve.

96. Grilled Apples with Cheese and Honey

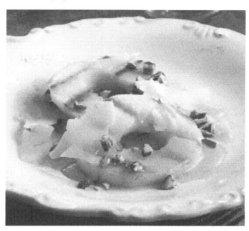

Nutritional values:

- Calories: 245
- Fat: 14 g
- Carbohydrate: 29.6 g
- Protein: 4.6 g

Ingredients:

- 1 small tart apple, peeled, cut into ½ inch thick round slices
- ½ teaspoon confectioners' sugar
- 1 tablespoon chopped pecans, toasted
- 1 teaspoon almond oil or canola oil
- ½ ounce cheddar cheese or parmesan cheese
- 2 teaspoons honey

Directions:

1. You can grill the apple on a preheated grill or in a grill pan.
2. If you are using the grill, set up your grill and preheat it to medium heat. In case you are using the grill pan, place the grill pan over medium heat and let it heat.
3. Place apple slices in a bowl. Drizzle oil over the apple slices and toss well.
4. Sprinkle sugar over the apple slices.
5. Place apples on the preheated grill or grill pan and cook for 3 minutes. Turn the apple slices over and cook the other side for 3 minutes.
6. Take out the apple slices from the grill and place on a plate.
7. Take a vegetable peeler and shave the cheese into strips. Place cheese strips over the apples.
8. Scatter pecans over the apples. Trickle honey on top and serve.

97. Avocado Ice Cream

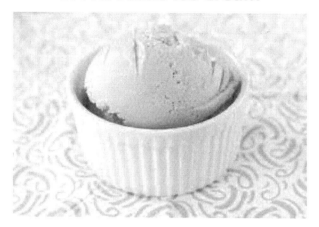

Nutritional values:

- Calories: 174
- Fat: 9 g
- Carbohydrate: 25 g
- Protein: 3 g

Ingredients:

- ¼ large banana, chop into chunks
- ¼ medium ripe avocado, peeled, pitted
- ½ cup frozen chopped mango
- ¼ cup unsweetened almond milk
- ½ cup raw spinach

Directions:

1. Place banana slices on a small tray and freeze until firm.
2. Add banana slices, almond milk, spinach, avocado, and mango in a blender and blend until smooth and creamy.
3. Transfer the blended mixture into a freezer safe container. Freeze until use.
4. Scoop the ice cream into a bowl and serve.

98. Strawberry Nice Cream

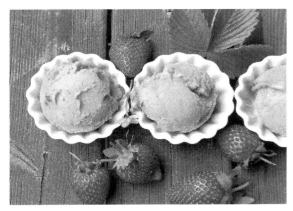

Nutritional values:

- Calories: 191

- Fat: 0.5 g

- Carbohydrate: 22.5 g

- Protein: 1.4 g

Ingredients:

- 4 ounces strawberries, hulled, coarsely chopped

- 1 tablespoon chilled water if required

- ¾ teaspoon fresh lemon juice

- 1 medium banana, peeled, coarsely chopped

Directions:

1. Take 2 small, freezer safe trays and spread the strawberries on one tray and banana on the other tray.

2. Place the trays in the freezer and freeze for a few hours until firm, about 8–10 hours.

3. Take out the tray with strawberries and keep it on your countertop for 15 minutes.

4. Place the strawberries in the food processor bowl and give short pulses until finely chopped.

5. Now add banana and lemon juice and process until creamy. Add chilled water if required while blending.

6. Scrape the sides of the bowl whenever required.

7. Serve right away if you want soft serve consistency. If you want firm, nice cream, pour into a freezer safe container and freeze for 30–45 minutes.

8. Serve.

99. Strawberry and Mango Sundae

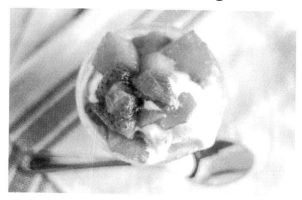

Nutritional values:

- Calories: 206
- Fat: 2.4 g
- Carbohydrate: 43.1 g
- Protein: 5.8 g

Ingredients:

- ¼ cup thawed frozen strawberries
- 1/8 teaspoon lemon juice or to taste
- ¼ mango, peeled, diced
- ½ tablespoon brown sugar
- 1 scoop nonfat vanilla frozen yogurt
- 1 tablespoon chopped toasted nuts

Directions:

1. Add strawberries, lemon juice, and sugar into a blender and blend until smooth.

2. Place the scoop of vanilla frozen yogurt in a dessert bowl.

3. Scatter mango and nuts in the bowl. Drizzle the blended strawberry mixture on top and serve.

100. Old—Fashioned Fruit Crumble for Two

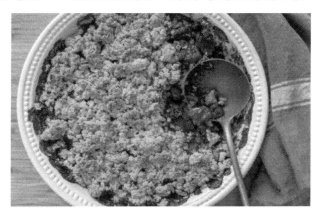

Nutritional values:

- Calories: 264
- Fat: 12.4 g
- Carbohydrate: 37.3 g
- Protein: 4.3 g

Ingredients:

- ¾ cup fresh or frozen fruit
- 2 teaspoons all-purpose flour, divided
- 1/8 cup old fashioned oats
- 2 teaspoons brown sugar
- ½ tablespoon canola oil
- ¾ teaspoon sugar
- ¾ teaspoon orange juice
- 1 ½ tablespoons chopped almonds
- 1/8 teaspoon ground cinnamon

Directions:

1. Set the temperature of your oven to 400 °F and preheat the oven.

2. Place fruit in a bowl. Add sugar, orange juice and ¾ teaspoon flour and mix well. Spoon the mixture into an ovenproof dish or ramekin.

3. Mix together brown sugar, almonds, oats, cinnamon and remaining flour in a bowl. Add oil and mix until well combined.

4. Scatter this mixture over the fruit, in the baking dish. Keep the baking dish on a baking sheet and place the baking sheet in the oven.

5. Bake for about 20 minutes or until golden brown on top.

WOULD YOU DO ME A FOVOR?

Thank you for reading my book.

I hope you'll use what you've learned to look, feel and live better than you ever have before.

I have a small favor to ask.

Would you mind taking a minute to write a blurb on Amazon about this book? I check all my reviews and love to get honest feedback.

That's the real pay for my work – knowing that I'm helping people.

>> Scan with your camera to leave a quick review:

Conclusion

It is never too late to focus on shifting to a healthier diet. What you eat plays a significant role in your overall health and sense of well-being. The proverbial saying which goes along the lines of, "You are what you eat," is in fact, true!

If you are struggling to shed those extra pounds, want a healthier eating pattern, or wish to achieve weight loss, the macro diet is ideal for you!

The macro diet is not like any regular and conventional diets. This diet is inclusive, varied, and can be customized as per your needs, requirements, and fitness or health objectives. The idea of this diet is incredibly simple. You must focus on consuming a healthy dose of the three macronutrients or macros your body requires — carbohydrates, proteins, and fats. As long as you cater to your body's needs and requirements, it will not let you down. This diet has taken the world of fitness and nutrition by storm and for all the right reasons. From making you more conscious of the foods you consume and teaching about wholesome nutrition to improving your overall health and sense of wellbeing, this diet has a lot to offer. What more? By now you would have realized how simple and effective this diet is. Also, all the results obtained from it are perfectly sustainable! Well, dieting certainly doesn't get any better or easier than this!

In this book, you were introduced to all the information required about understanding the macro diet. From what it means to all the benefits it offers and the protocols it entails, this book will act as your guide every step of the way. Whether you want to lose fat, maintain weight loss, develop lean muscle, or simply consume well-balanced meals, tracking your macros is needed. Tracking macros probably sounds slightly complicated but it is not. With the right information doing this is incredibly simple. In this book, you were given all the information required to follow this diet. From helping you understand the importance of macronutrients to the nutritional profile of some common ingredients you consume; this book has a lot to offer. You were also introduced to simple steps that can be followed to understand your daily calorie and macronutrient requirements based on your goals.

This book also gives you the needed suggestions to understand how to adjust the macros, sample meal plans, and tips to create a meal plan that fits your needs and requirements. What more? It also includes a variety of recipes that will make it easier to follow the macro diet. The recipes given in this book are divided into different categories for your convenience. They're not only easy and simple to cook but are extremely nutritious and tasty as well. Regardless of your level of cooking skills or the time available, you can find recipes that cater to your needs and requirements. Getting used to counting and tracking macros takes time and effort. However, the little effort you make initially will pay off later. Once you get into the groove of it, you will be able to do it automatically!

All it requires is careful consideration, some planning, commitment, and some conscious effort. Once you are willing to do all this, achieving your weight loss and health goals becomes a perfectly achievable and maintainable goal. So, what are you waiting for? Now that you are armed with the right information, the next step is to simply get started! The key to your health and well-being lies in your hands. There is no time like the present to regain this control and live the best life possible!

FREE BONUS MATERIAL

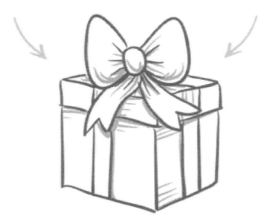

Thank you for reading this book. I hope you find it insightful, inspiring, and practical and I hope it helps you build that strong and healthy body you really desire.

To help you get the best results as fast as possible I've put together additional free resources:

- **Macro Friendly Grocery List** to never run out of ideas what to eat
- **6 Step Quick Start Guide** to finally take your fitness under control
- **Daily Checklist** to stay on track with your fitness goals
- **Example Meal Plan** to supercharge your fat loss
- **Comprehensive Workout Log Sheet** for keeping track of your workouts
- **Top Tips for Seniors** to enjoy your life and avoid health problems as you age

To get your bonuses go to:
http://bit.ly/4oMJRRK

or scan QR code with your camera

At **BODY YOU DESERVE Publishing**, we strongly believe that there are a thousand ways to improve your life and health. However, there is no single recipe suitable for everyone how to do that.

We think that the best way to receive your goals is the one you can stick to and our writers will do their best to provide simple, easy to follow, step by step and realistic instructions how to do that.

To discover our best books go to link:

https://amzn.to/40B5KmZ

Or scan QR code with your camera:

References

American College of Sports Medicine (2015). *Protein intake for optimal muscle maintenance.* https://www.acsm.org/docs/default-source/files-for-resource-library/protein-intake-for-optimal-muscle-maintenance.pdf

Capritto, A. (n.d.). *How to calculate and track your macronutrients.* CNET. https://www.cnet.com/health/nutrition/ultimate-guide-to-counting-and-tracking-macros/

Dresden, D. (2020, April 21). *How does alcohol affect weight loss? What to know.* Medical News Today. https://www.medicalnewstoday.com/articles/alcohol-and-weight-loss#tips

How to calculate TDEE (Total Daily Energy Expenditure). (n.d.). Opex Fit. https://www.opexfit.com/blog/how-to-calculate-tdee-total-daily-energy-expenditure

If it fits your macros: You need to know the truth. (2017, March 27). U.P. Blog. https://blog.ultimateperformance.com/if-it-fits-your-macros-you-need-to-know-the-truth/#:~:text=You%27ve%20probably%20heard%20of

Julson, E. (2018, June 5). *IIFYM (If It Fits Your Macros): A beginner's guide.* Healthline. https://www.healthline.com/nutrition/iifym-guide#:~:text=Adjust%20based%20on%20weight%20goals

Kittman, B. (2019, May 13). *5 benefits of tracking your macros | SD Entertainer Magazine.* San Diego Entertainment Magazine. Https://www.sdentertainer.com/lifestyle/5-benefits-of-tracking-your-macros/

Matthews, M. (2014). Bigger Leaner Stronger: The Simple Science of Building the Ultimate Male Body. In *Amazon* (3rd edition). Oculus Publishers. https://www.amazon.com/Bigger-Leaner-Stronger-Building-Ultimate-ebook/dp/B006XF5BTG

Macronutrients: A simple guide to macros. (2019, September 5). Avita Health System. https://avitahealth.org/health-library/macronutrients-a-simple-guide-to-macros/

McGuire, S. (2011). U.S. Department of Agriculture and U.S. Department of Health and Human Services, Dietary Guidelines for Americans, 2010. 7th Edition, Washington, DC: U.S. Government Printing Office, January 2011. *Advances in Nutrition*, *2*(3), 293–294. https://doi.org/10.3945/an.111.000430

Wempen, K. (2022, April 29). *Are you getting too much protein*. Mayo Clinic Health System. https://www.mayoclinichealthsystem.org/hometown-health/speaking-of-health/are-you-getting-too-much-protein

References for Images

Braxmeier, H. (2014, January 3). *Potato soup* [Pixabay]. https://pixabay.com/photos/potato-soup-mashed-potatoes-237760/

Breen, D. (2015, December 8). *Breakfast parfait* [Pixabay]. https://pixabay.com/photos/yogurt-parfait-glass-fruit-fresh-1081135/

congerdesign. (2021, June 17). *Banana and almond butter oatmeal* [Pixabay]. https://pixabay.com/photos/muesli-oatmeal-breakfast-healthy-6342969/

ElodiV. (2017, August 17). *Chocolate mousse* [Pixabay]. https://pixabay.com/photos/chocolate-mousse-aquafaba-vegan-2635501/

ExplorerBob. (2017, August 15). *Cranberry vanilla oatmeal* [Pixabay]. https://pixabay.com/photos/oatmeal-dried-cranberries-2645945/

kakuko. (2016, May 3). *Sautéed broccoli stir fry recipe with garlic* [Pixabay]. https://pixabay.com/photos/wok-dish-asian-rice-meal-chinese-1363477/

Lipinski, M. (2018, October 11). *Lentil sausage stew* [Pixabay]. https://pixabay.com/photos/lentil-soup-lenses-stew-food-3738547/

Mehta, S. (2020, April 2). *Pita pepperoni pizza* [Pixabay]. https://pixabay.com/photos/pepperoni-pizza-thin-crest-4991789/

nemoelguedes. (2015, May 21). *Tomato basil omelet* [Pixabay]. https://pixabay.com/photos/kitchen-omelet-eggs-food-healthy-775746/

pixel2013. (2018, March 10). *Green eggs* [Pixabay]. https://pixabay.com/photos/food-meal-spinach-fried-egg-yummy-3214904/

RitaE. (2018, August 30). *Steak* [Pixabay]. https://pixabay.com/photos/steak-meat-beef-steak-food-beef-3640560/

silviarita. (2017, April 18). *Strawberry nice cream* [Pixabay]. https://pixabay.com/photos/strawberry-ice-cream-strawberries-2239377/

Steinert, T. (2017, March 5). *White bean turkey chili* [Pixabay]. https://pixabay.com/photos/food-stew-chili-con-carne-meal-2112302/

StockSnap. (2017, August 6). *Chocolate brownie* [Pixabay]. https://pixabay.com/photos/dessert-food-chocolate-brownie-2603520/

Sylvester, M. (2016, September 15). *Devilled eggs* [Pixabay]. https://pixabay.com/photos/home-cooking-deviled-eggs-eggs-1670403/

tomwieden. (2021, April 30). *Healthy mashed sweet potatoes* [Pixabay]. https://pixabay.com/photos/mashed-sweet-potato-food-dish-meal-6218759/

Towner, C. (2015, December 30). *Greek couscous salad* [Pixabay]. https://pixabay.com/photos/couscous-vegetables-tomatoes-dinner-1112012/

valero. (2021, August 13). *Black bean quesadillas* [Pixabay]. https://pixabay.com/photos/quesadillas-food-mexico-6539731/

Valencia, J. (2017, February 26). *Shrimp pad thai* [Pixabay]. https://pixabay.com/photos/pad-thai-noodles-thai-pad-asian-2098017/

Wachman, O. (2019, September 24). *Baked spicy chicken wings* [Pixabay]. https://pixabay.com/photos/food-chicken-wings-chicken-4497587/

15538942R00108